Student Workbook and Resource Guide for

# Medical–Surgical Nursing Care

Fourth Edition

Karen M. Burke, RN, MS
Elaine L. Mohn-Brown, RN, EdD
Linda Eby, RN, MN

**PEARSON**

Boston   Columbus   Indianapolis   New York   San Francisco   Hoboken   Amsterdam
Cape Town   Dubai   London   Madrid   Milan   Munich   Paris   Montréal   Toronto   Delhi
Mexico City   São Paulo   Sydney   Hong Kong   Seoul   Singapore   Taipei   Tokyo

Pearson® is a registered trademark of Pearson plc

Pearson Education LTD.
Pearson Education Australia PTY, Limited
Pearson Education Singapore, Pte. Ltd
Pearson Education North Asia Ltd
Pearson Education, Canada, Ltd

Pearson Educación de Mexico, S.A. de C.V.
Pearson Education—Japan
Pearson Education Malaysia, Pte. Ltd
Pearson Education, Hoboken, New Jersey

**PEARSON**

10 9 8 7 6 5 4 3 2 1

ISBN 10:     0-134-00432-9

ISBN 13: 978-0-134-00432-7

# Contents

# Preface

Students entering the field of nursing have a tremendous amount to learn in a very short time. This concise student workbook and resource guide has been developed to help you learn and apply key concepts and procedures and master critical-thinking skills based on *Medical–Surgical Nursing Care.*

Each chapter includes a variety of questions and activities to help you comprehend difficult concepts and reinforce basic knowledge gained from textbook reading assignments. Highlights of this workbook include:

- Chapters that correlate directly to *Medical–Surgical Nursing Care* to allow you to easily locate information related to each question.
- Thorough assessment of essential information in the chapter through generous use of multiple-choice and matching-style questions.
- Clinical case studies that provide scenarios to sharpen critical-thinking and clinical reasoning skills.
- Answers included in an appendix to provide immediate reinforcement and to allow you to check the accuracy of your work.

It is our hope that this workbook contributes to your success in the exciting and challenging field of medical–surgical nursing care.

# CHAPTER 1

# Nursing in the 21st Century

## KEY TERMS

Match each term with its appropriate definition.

1. Patient-centered care
2. Caregivers
3. Advocate
4. Holistic
5. Assessment
6. Nursing diagnosis
7. Outcomes
8. Critical thinking
9. Standard
10. Malpractice

A. Concerned with the whole person—physical, emotional, spiritual aspects

B. First phase of the nursing process

C. People who provide personal assistance

D. Conclusion about a patient's health status

E. Use of cognitive knowledge to choose best action

F. Criterion to measure quality of practice

G. Harm that results through actions of a licensed person

H. Care focused on the uniqueness of the individual

I. Achievable, measurable goals

J. One who speaks for another and promotes patient's rights

## LEARNING OUTCOMES

1. What is medical–surgical nursing?
2. Describe four ways nurses promote and provide care to adult patients.
3. What is quality improvement?
4. What are some objectives of an advocate?
5. List the phases of the nursing process.
6. What is critical thinking?
7. Name five roles of the LPN/LVN in medical–surgical nursing practice.
8. What is the purpose of HIPAA?
9. Define *ethics*.
10. What are professional boundaries?

# APPLY WHAT YOU LEARNED

The student nurses are beginning to study the nursing process. The students understand that the process is individualized and begins with data collection.

1. Describe the phases of the nursing process.
2. What happens during the evaluation phase?
3. Why is selecting a nursing diagnosis an important part of the process?

# MULTIPLE CHOICE

Circle the answer that best completes the following statements.

1. A choice between two unpleasant alternatives is known as:
   A. ethics.
   B. assessment.
   C. dilemma.
   D. evaluation.

2. The ethical principle that involves the nurse avoiding doing harm to patients is:
   A. beneficence.
   B. autonomy.
   C. accountability.
   D. nonmaleficence.

3. Purposeful actions to meet physical, psychosocial, and cultural needs of patients are:
   A. interventions.
   B. quality assurance.
   C. nursing diagnosis.
   D. implementation.

4. Nursing that is concerned with the whole person—physical, emotional, and spiritual—is:
   A. medical.
   B. psychologic.
   C. ethical.
   D. holistic.

5. The nurse is teaching the patient about a medication that has just been prescribed. Review of side effects and length of treatment has the patient concerned. The nurse knows that giving the patient this information to make decisions regarding care makes the nurse an:
   A. ethics committee member.
   B. advocate.
   C. implementation specialist.
   D. identifier of data.

6. Medical information that is obtained through observation or measurement is known as:

   **A.** objective.

   **B.** subjective.

   **C.** data.

   **D.** focused.

7. The nurse recognizes that designing interventions and outcomes is part of which phase of the nursing process?

   **A.** Diagnosis

   **B.** Implementation

   **C.** Assessment

   **D.** Planning

8. Determining whether the plan was effective or needs to be revised is completed during:

   **A.** evaluation.

   **B.** implementation.

   **C.** planning.

   **D.** assessing.

9. Recognizing a pattern or clinical situation and combining it with knowledge and previous experience is known as:

   **A.** empathy.

   **B.** discipline.

   **C.** intuition.

   **D.** intellectual courage.

10. Laws that limit nursing practice to those licensed and practicing as nurses within a state are known as:

    **A.** scope of practice.

    **B.** statutory law.

    **C.** regulatory law.

    **D.** administrative law.

11. The nurse going to the cafeteria with friends begins to tell them about a new patient. The nurse says that the patient is her mother's neighbor and continues to discuss his medical care. The nurse should understand that this is a violation of:

    **A.** ethics.

    **B.** malpractice.

    **C.** HIPAA.

    **D.** standards.

12. When a nurse administers a medication against the will of a mentally competent patient, it is known as:

    **A.** battery.

    **B.** assault.

    **C.** defamation.

    **D.** false imprisonment.

13. Managing and using data, information, and knowledge through computer information systems is:
    A. quality assurance.
    B. risk management.
    C. informatics.
    D. health care informatics.

14. The phase of the nursing process that includes a thorough history and physical assessment is:
    A. initial assessment.
    B. objective data.
    C. subjective data.
    D. focused assessment.

15. The nurse understands that using knowledge, experience, understanding, values, and ability to identify options is part of which process?
    A. Ethical dilemmas
    B. Clinical reasoning
    C. Intuition
    D. Planning

# CHAPTER 2 ▸ Health, Illness, and Settings of Care

## KEY TERMS

Match each term with its appropriate definition.

1. Health
2. Homeostasis
3. Disease
4. Manifestations
5. Illness
6. Acute illness
7. Remission
8. Acuity
9. Chronic illness
10. Rehabilitation

A. Maintaining a dynamic steady state or balance

B. Signs and symptoms

C. Disease that occurs rapidly and is self-limiting

D. The severity of illness and level of care required

E. Disruptions in the structure and function of the body or mind

F. Condition that requires continuing management over a long period

G. Process of achieving one's maximum potential after acute illness

H. Period in which the patient is not experiencing symptoms even though disease is present

I. Response a person has to a disease

J. State of complete physical, mental, and social well-being

## LEARNING OUTCOMES

1. What is the health–illness continuum?
2. List some leading health indicators for *Healthy People 2020*.
3. What is illness?
4. Name five characteristics of a chronic illness.
5. What is long-term care?
6. What is community-based nursing?
7. Name eight or more community-based nursing care settings.
8. What patients benefit from home health care services?
9. List safety concerns a home health nurse should assess.
10. Name five suggestions for effective home care.

# APPLY WHAT YOU LEARNED

The nurse is assigned to care for a 72-year-old patient who has been experiencing falls and some cognitive issues. Upon entering the patient's home, the nurse notices that the bathroom is on the second floor, and the house appears dark and poorly lit.

1. What safety issues should the nurse teach the patient?
2. What community resources could the nurse recommend?

# MULTIPLE CHOICE

Circle the answer that best completes the following statements.

1. The body's tendency to maintain a dynamic steady state or balance under constantly changing conditions is:
   A. homeostasis.
   B. disease.
   C. illness.
   D. wellness.

2. A disease that can spread from one person to another is known as:
   A. congenital.
   B. idiopathic.
   C. communicable.
   D. latrogenic.

3. The nurse understands that the purpose of community-based care is to provide direct services to individuals to manage health problems and promote:
   A. nursing.
   B. medicine.
   C. physicians.
   D. self-care.

4. The process of learning to live to one's maximum potential with a chronic impairment and the resulting functional disability is known as:
   A. long-term care.
   B. disability.
   C. rehabilitation.
   D. cognitive therapy.

5. The nurse is caring for a patient who presents with pain, nausea, and anxiety. These are known as:
   A. assessments.
   B. stressors.
   C. manifestations.
   D. disease.

6. A patient has been undergoing testing for complaints of abdominal pain. All tests have come back negative, and the patient is still experiencing pain. The nurse knows the class of disease with an unknown cause is known as:

   A. congenital.

   B. psychosomatic.

   C. iatrogenic.

   D. idiopathic.

7. A period of time where symptoms reappear during an illness is:

   A. exacerbation.

   B. remission.

   C. end stage.

   D. acute.

8. The severity of the patient's illness and level of care required is referred to as:

   A. illness.

   B. acuity.

   C. disease.

   D. health care continuum.

9. The nurse is doing a home evaluation for a 72-year-old patient who lives alone. What would indicate an intervention by the nurse?

   A. Current medications

   B. Inadequate food supply

   C. Absence of throw rugs

   D. Open blinds

10. The purpose of a home health care nurse's nursing assessment visit is to:

    A. formulate a diagnosis for the physician.

    B. submit to Medicare.

    C. refer to the nursing home.

    D. identify the patient's needs.

11. The nurse understands that all of the following are community-based nursing care settings EXCEPT:

    A. mental health centers.

    B. senior centers.

    C. hospitals.

    D. free clinics.

12. A nurse who helps to bridge gaps between members of the church and the health care system is involved in:

    A. mental health nursing.

    B. home health nursing.

    C. forensic nursing.

    D. parish nursing.

13. The degree of observable and measurable impairment is known as:
   A. impairment.
   B. handicap.
   C. rehabilitation.
   D. disability.

14. A chronic illness is characterized by all of the following EXCEPT it:
   A. is permanent.
   B. leaves a disability.
   C. is reversible.
   D. requires long periods of care.

15. The nurse understands that an acute illness is:
   A. nonreversible.
   B. self-limiting.
   C. malignant.
   D. congenital.

# CHAPTER 3

# Cultural and Developmental Considerations for Adults

## KEY TERMS

Match each term with its appropriate definition.

1. Culture
2. Race
3. Personal space
4. Alterations in health
5. Family
6. Ethnic group
7. Ethnocentrism
8. Nuclear family
9. Health disparities
10. Extended families

A. Area surrounding one's body
B. Change from the normal health state
C. Learned behavior started by a group of people
D. Group of people who share backgrounds such as religion or residence
E. Peoples' beliefs that their values are the only acceptable ones
F. Multigenerational family unit, including all relatives
G. Differences in health outcomes that occur among specific population groups
H. Man, woman, and biological children
I. Unit of people related by marriage, birth, or adoption
J. Differences in physical characteristics, such as skin color and eye shape

## LEARNING OUTCOMES

1. Name five components of culture.
2. What are health disparities?
3. What special care considerations are there for Jehovah's Witnesses?
4. List health risks for young adults.
5. What are the tasks of a family?
6. Why is culturally sensitive care important for nurses?
7. List three differences in health behaviors of the young adult and middle adult.
8. What importance does personal space have?
9. What is social orientation?
10. Identify some health risks for middle adults.

# APPLY WHAT YOU LEARNED

The student nurse is speaking with high school students regarding growth and development. Some students tell her that they have one father and a stepmother, while other students report having lived with grandparents or two mothers.

1. What types of family structures are represented?
2. What types of health promotion could be taught to these students?

# MULTIPLE CHOICE

Circle the answer that best completes the following statements.

1. A group of people who share experiences and backgrounds based on status, religion, and residence is known as the:
   A. cultural group.
   B. race group.
   C. social group.
   D. ethnic group.

2. The nurse knows that the middle adult is within the age range of:
   A. 65–85.
   B. 36–60.
   C. 25–55.
   D. 40–65.

3. When speaking to a group of women between 18 and 40, the nurse knows the importance of a clinic breast exam at least every:
   A. 3 years.
   B. 5 years.
   C. 1 year.
   D. 2 years.

4. When providing culturally competent care, the nurse must:
   A. have a detailed understanding of the beliefs and values of all his or her patients.
   B. accept and respect differences in his or her patients.
   C. follow his or her own personal beliefs when assessing patients.
   D. be judgmental.

5. The nurse is teaching a patient about personal space. Knowing this patient is from Latin America means that the patient requires:
   A. more personal space.
   B. less personal space.
   C. no personal space.
   D. eye contact only.

6. A Roman Catholic patient is having his first post-op meal on Friday and the nurse is helping him select his menu. Considering Lent, which food should be avoided?

   **A.** Broccoli

   **B.** Milk

   **C.** Hamburger

   **D.** Salmon

7. To give the most culturally competent care, the nurse must be aware of:

   **A.** psychology.

   **B.** his or her own values.

   **C.** anatomy.

   **D.** physiology.

8. *Temporal orientation* means:

   **A.** sound judgment.

   **B.** balanced thoughts.

   **C.** orientation in time.

   **D.** future judgment.

9. Recognizing the denomination of Seventh-Day Adventist, the nurse needs to respect that this day is considered the Sabbath for them:

   **A.** Monday

   **B.** Saturday

   **C.** Sunday

   **D.** Friday

10. The nurse recognizes that the beginning of wrinkles, gray hair, decreased gastric secretions, and some loss of visual acuity occurs starting in the:

    **A.** 20s.

    **B.** 30s.

    **C.** 40s.

    **D.** 50s.

11. The leading cause of injury and death in people between ages 15 and 44 is:

    **A.** accidents.

    **B.** suicide.

    **C.** occupational.

    **D.** homicides.

12. When considering the most widely used drug among young adults, the nurse would know that it is:

    **A.** cocaine.

    **B.** alcohol.

    **C.** marijuana.

    **D.** heroin.

13. What degree of change in glucose tolerance occurs in the middle adult?
    A. None
    B. Gradual decrease
    C. Gradual increase
    D. Sudden decrease

14. A unit of people related by marriage, birth, or adoption is called a:
    A. family.
    B. culture.
    C. ethnic group.
    D. race.

15. The nurse understands that by promoting health in adult patients through education, he or she is also promoting:
    A. nursing.
    B. community.
    C. wellness.
    D. faith.

# CHAPTER 4

# The Older Adult in Health and Illness

## KEY TERMS

Match each term with its appropriate definition.

1. Geriatrics
2. Cognition
3. Widowhood
4. Gerontologic nursing
5. Ageism
6. Dementia
7. Reminiscence
8. Senescence
9. Sundowning syndrome
10. Falls

A. The older adult becomes confused and agitated after dark

B. Term used to refer to different kinds of organic disorders that progressively affect cognitive function

C. Most common cause of injuries to older adults

D. Aging

E. Life review; when adults tell stories of their past

F. Loss of a spouse

G. Form of prejudice against older adults

H. Area of health care that focuses on the holistic care of older adults

I. Nursing care of the older adult

J. Ability to perceive and understand one's world

## LEARNING OUTCOMES

1. Define *ageism*, and list two myths about older adults.
2. What is gerontologic nursing, and what is the projected future of this trend?
3. Discuss the term *cognition*, and list some examples pertaining to the older adult.
4. Which developmental stage does Erikson identify for the older adult?
5. How would the nurse encourage reminiscence in the older adult?
6. What are some age-related physical changes in the older adult?
7. What is meant by psychosocial change? List some examples.
8. How would the nurse teach the older adult about prevention of accidents?
9. What is Alzheimer disease?
10. How would the nurse describe methods to improve or maintain an older adult's quality of life?

## APPLY WHAT YOU LEARNED

You are working with a patient who is about to be discharged from the hospital after a fall. She will be returning to her home, where she lives alone. She is 68 years old and takes medication only for hypertension. Her family is present at the time of discharge and tells you that they will stop over and check on her periodically.

1. What are some teaching points you can give to the patient and family about preventing accidents in the home?
2. What are some concepts that will assist in the health promotion of the older adult?
3. Would you request other disciplines to see her? If so, why?

## MULTIPLE CHOICE

Circle the answer that best completes the following statements.

1. The nurse overhears a 76-year-old patient's family member state, "Well he's had his good years. What can he possibly do to help us when he gets out?" This is a form of:
   A. genetic theory.
   B. apoptosis.
   C. ageism.
   D. senescence.

2. Calcium intake in older adults should average:
   A. 1,200 mg/day.
   B. 600 mg/day.
   C. 800 mg/day.
   D. 1,600 mg/day.

3. Older people continue to develop:
   A. judgmentally.
   B. intelligence.
   C. gerontologically.
   D. accidentally.

4. You are assessing the physical condition of an 80-year-old male. You will not be surprised to find which of these signs and symptoms?
   A. Rales
   B. Decreased skin turgor
   C. Smooth skin
   D. Visual acuity of 20/20

5. When making a home visit to your 66-year-old patient, she states, "I made fried chicken and a peach cobbler yesterday. Would you care for some?" Your best reply should be:
   A. "Oh, no, that's too much fat!"
   B. "Sure, where is the butter?"
   C. "I will send a dietician to discuss alternative cooking options."
   D. "Did you make collard greens also?"

6. The nurse is teaching the daughter of an older patient about the aging process. The nurse would be correct if she stated:

   A. "Your father may develop an enlarged prostate."

   B. "Estrogen levels begin to increase in females as they get older."

   C. "Hypoglycemia is common in the older adult."

   D. "Infection risks are decreased due to the adrenal gland's enlargement."

7. Which of the following conditions would most likely be seen in the older adult?

   A. Cataracts

   B. Hypotension

   C. Herpes

   D. Obesity

8. You are talking to a patient's son about the care his 78-year-old father will need at home. Your greatest concern for this patient should be:

   A. risk for falls.

   B. risk for infection.

   C. risk for impaired mobility.

   D. risk for caregiver-role strain.

9. The nurse is aware that a family that takes care of a patient with Alzheimer disease:

   A. realizes the disease is reversible.

   B. allows the patient to wander without constraint.

   C. may need the help of a support group.

   D. provides a stimulating environment.

10. Illness and loss of independence are:

    A. an expected part of the aging process.

    B. not inevitable.

    C. government issues.

    D. all of the above.

11. Depression is often confused with:

    A. confusion.

    B. seizures.

    C. dementia.

    D. dehydration.

12. When evaluating the nutritional status of an older patient, the nurse should be especially aware of:

    A. exercise routine.

    B. environmental factors.

    C. lost or damaged teeth/dentures.

    D. fiber intake.

13. The nurse knows that the following teaching methods can be adapted for older adults:

    **A.** speaking more loudly.

    **B.** using simpler words.

    **C.** providing written material and using charts and literature with large print.

    **D.** explaining that getting older is associated with confusion.

14. In understanding the genitourinary system of the older adult, the nurse knows:

    **A.** kidneys increase in mass.

    **B.** kidneys decrease in mass.

    **C.** micturition reflex is increased.

    **D.** bladder capacity increases.

15. To assist older adults in reminiscence, the nurse would ask:

    **A.** open-ended questions.

    **B.** yes/no questions so as to not confuse them.

    **C.** them to remember numerous details.

    **D.** them about painful memories.

# CHAPTER 5

# Guidelines for Patient Assessment

## KEY TERMS

Match each term with its appropriate definition.

1. Inspection
2. Palpation
3. Percussion
4. Auscultation
5. Subjective data
6. Objective data
7. Dyspnea
8. Orthopnea
9. Manifestations
10. Assessment

A. Signs; observable or measurable information

B. Tapping the body to produce sound waves

C. Breathing more easily in an upright position

D. Observing/looking carefully

E. Symptoms experienced by the patient

F. Listening to sounds using a stethoscope

G. Difficulty breathing

H. Objective and subjective data associated with an illness

I. Using the hands to touch and feel

J. Process of collecting data that provide information about the patient's health care needs

## LEARNING OUTCOMES

1. What are the three purposes of the patient assessment?
2. What are the differences between subjective and objective data?
3. List components in a health history.
4. List four methods of physical examination.
5. What are some age-related assessment findings in the older adult?
6. Describe the assessment of the pupils.
7. Compare bradycardia and tachycardia.
8. What are the two sources of assessment data? Which is the best source?
9. How does the nurse evaluate mental status?
10. What are the key concepts in documenting accurately?

# APPLY WHAT YOU LEARNED

A patient presents to your clinic with complaints of general body aches, little joy in activities, and loss of appetite. You notice the patient is wearing torn clothes and appears unkempt. Through initial conversation, you discover that the patient is a 34-year-old recently unemployed male who has two children to support.

1. Based on this scenario, what type of data would be considered objective?
2. Could the nurse list subjective data based on the given information?
3. What type of assessment would the nurse focus on?

# MULTIPLE CHOICE

Circle the answer that best completes the following statements.

1. Poor turgor and dry mucous membranes would be an indication of:
   A. fluid volume deficit.
   B. fluid volume excess.
   C. normal fluid balance.
   D. acid–base excess.

2. A grating sound heard during chest auscultation may be:
   A. crackles.
   B. pleural friction rub.
   C. rhonchi.
   D. wheezes.

3. Your patient complains of difficulty breathing when attempting to lie down. After your respiratory assessment, you see in the medical record that the patient has a history of:
   A. eupnea.
   B. apnea.
   C. orthopnea.
   D. dyspnea.

4. After the assessment of the eyes, the nurse would not document:
   A. equality.
   B. shape.
   C. reactivity.
   D. color of iris.

5. The normal pupillary response to accommodation is:
   A. dilatation and divergence.
   B. dilatation and constriction.
   C. constriction and divergence.
   D. constriction and convergence.

6. The use of adequate lighting is most important during:

   A. auscultation.

   B. percussion.

   C. palpation.

   D. inspection.

7. Ms. Lewis has a fractured tibia and fibula. The nurse is performing an assessment of her extremities. The purpose of squeezing the patient's fingernail is to evaluate:

   A. peripheral circulation.

   B. cardiac output.

   C. peripheral pulses.

   D. nutritional deficiencies.

8. The student nurse is performing a cardiac assessment and finds the patient's pulse rate is 130 beats per minute. The nurse understands that a common cause of tachycardia is:

   A. bright lights.

   B. sputum production.

   C. pain and anxiety.

   D. cyanosis.

9. While assessing your patient's lung fields, you hear popping sounds during inspiration at the base of the left lung. You would classify these findings as:

   A. crackles.

   B. rhonchi.

   C. wheezes.

   D. rubs.

10. An example of objective data would include:

    A. the patient's description of the pain.

    B. radial pulse rate of 66 beats per minute.

    C. sensation of itching after a bee sting.

    D. headache resulting from photosensitivity.

11. A patient states that he has had severe abdominal cramping for the last 2 hours. This type of data would be classified as an example of:

    A. subjective data.

    B. objective data.

    C. disputable data.

    D. personal data.

12. When assessing peripheral pulses, the nurse must compare both extremities. The elements of this assessment include:

    A. rate.

    B. rhythm.

    C. strength.

    D. all of the above.

13. The nurse prepares to assess the patient's abdomen. The correct order of assessment should be:

    A. inspection, auscultation, palpation.

    B. inspection, palpation, auscultation.

    C. auscultation, inspection, palpation.

    D. any order is acceptable.

14. Mr. Hibbard has been admitted to the orthopedic unit following a motor vehicle crash. Both arms are placed in long-arm casts. When taking the vital signs, the nurse must assess the pulse rate by:

    A. listening to the apical pulse for one full minute.

    B. placing the patient on a cardiac monitor.

    C. checking the carotid pulses.

    D. not assessing the radial pulses due to the location of the cast.

15. The most accurate method for assessing the pulse rate is:

    A. simultaneous bilateral manipulation of the carotid arteries.

    B. auscultating the apical pulse.

    C. palpating the radial pulses.

    D. auscultating the femoral pulses.

## KEY TERMS

Match each term with its appropriate definition.

1. Pharmacology
2. Pharmacokinetics
3. Biotransformation
4. Loading dose
5. Sentinel event
6. Synergism
7. Additive
8. Potentiation
9. Antagonist
10. Half-life

A. An initial higher-than-normal dose of the drug

B. The study of drugs and their uses in the body

C. Effect that develops when two drugs with similar actions are taken

D. Drug metabolism

E. Drug that prevents a receptor response or blocks a normal cellular response

F. When two drugs given together cause a greater response than each drug given separately

G. Any unexpected event in a health care facility that causes death or serious injury

H. Process by which the action of one drug increases the effect of the second drug

I. The amount of time needed for elimination processes to decrease the original blood concentration by 50%

J. The study of how drugs are processed by the body

## LEARNING OUTCOMES

1. What are the six rights of medication administration?
2. Describe the process of absorption and excretion in pharmacology.
3. What are the four names given to drugs?
4. What is the purpose of a loading dose?
5. Identify the differences between an idiosyncratic effect and a toxic effect.
6. Contrast agonist and antagonist drugs.
7. What is polypharmacy?
8. List some factors that affect drug responses.
9. Describe the concepts of synergism and potentiation.
10. List some factors to include in a medication history.

## APPLY WHAT YOU LEARNED

You are caring for a 65-year-old male who tells you that he takes five prescription drugs and three over-the-counter medications that his physician is not aware he is taking. As the nurse, you begin to educate the patient about the importance of reporting all medications to the physician.

1. Describe some educational points the nurse will address with this patient.
2. How will the nurse relay this information to the physician?
3. Discuss polypharmacy regarding this patient.

## MULTIPLE CHOICE

Circle the answer that best completes the following statements.

1. All health care facilities are required to have narcotic control systems in place (i.e., all narcotics are locked up). One way of ensuring compliance is to:
   A. give narcotic keys to all employees.
   B. give narcotic keys to administrative staff only.
   C. give narcotic keys to authorized personnel.
   D. not provide patients with narcotics.

2. The most readily available and accurate sources of drug information are:
   A. textbooks.
   B. *Micromedex* and *Hospital Formulary.*
   C. FDA and EPA.
   D. websites.

3. The absorption process occurs from the time a drug enters the body until:
   A. it reaches the site of action.
   B. half-life is achieved.
   C. excretion.
   D. it quits working.

4. Transdermal (applied to the skin) patches allow the body to absorb drugs slowly and usually:
   A. last longer.
   B. fall off easily.
   C. cause rashes.
   D. provide relief.

5. Intravenous drugs are delivered directly into the bloodstream and therefore have the:
   A. slowest excretion rate.
   B. fastest absorption rate.
   C. greatest half-life.
   D. longest duration of action.

6. The blood–brain barrier protects the central nervous system against severe toxic drug effects by preventing access to the:
   A. spinal fluid.
   B. cerebrospinal fluid.
   C. synovial fluid.
   D. pleural cavity.

7. *Drug metabolism* refers to the process by which the body changes a drug from its original chemical structure to a form that can be readily eliminated or excreted. This is also called:
   A. biochemistry.
   B. bionics.
   C. biotransformation.
   D. bioefficiency.

8. Drug toxicity in older adults occurs as a result of:
   A. ageism.
   B. negligence.
   C. confusion.
   D. polypharmacy.

9. The effect of a drug depends on its:
   A. type and patient.
   B. time and route.
   C. action and dose.
   D. cost and manufacturer.

10. The nurse knows to include in her teaching that:
    A. teas bind with tetracycline.
    B. a high-carbohydrate diet decreases the absorption of levodopa.
    C. a diet high in vitamin K reduces the effect of warfarin.
    D. a diet low in protein delays the effect of theophylline.

11. The usual adult dose of a drug is based on which body weight?
    A. 200 pound
    B. 100 kg
    C. 150 pound
    D. 150 kg

12. Over-the-counter (OTC) drugs account for what percentage of medication?
    A. 20
    B. 60
    C. 50
    D. 80

13. What does the nurse check before administering any drug?
    A. Allergies
    B. Likes and dislikes
    C. Side effects on the mother
    D. Insurance information

14. Which of these would not be included in a medication history?
    A. Allergies
    B. Use of OTC drugs
    C. Financial resources
    D. Employment status

15. What is the most important factor in administering medications to a 4-year-old child?
    A. Weight of the child
    B. Age of the child
    C. Ethnicity of the child
    D. Sex of the child

# CHAPTER 7 ▶ Caring for Patients With Altered Fluid, Electrolyte, or Acid–Base Balance

## KEY TERMS

Match each term with its appropriate definition.

1. Dehydration
2. Intracellular fluid
3. Edema
4. Extracellular fluid
5. Hypervolemia
6. Dyspnea
7. Hypoxemia
8. Respiratory acidosis
9. Electrolytes
10. Fluid volume deficit

A. Substances that separate in solution to form electrically charged particles
B. Commonly caused by diarrhea or vomiting
C. Excess fluid in body tissue
D. Occurs when carbon dioxide is retained
E. Fluid found outside the cells
F. Difficult or labored breathing
G. Low oxygen levels in the arterial blood
H. Fluid found inside the cells
I. May occur due to excessive fluid losses, insufficient fluid intake, or both
J. Excess intravascular fluid

## LEARNING OUTCOMES

1. Contrast intracellular and extracellular fluid.
2. What are the vital functions of water in the body?
3. What is the purpose of electrolytes?
4. List components of body fluid regulation.
5. What are some causes of fluid volume deficit?
6. What are some causes of fluid volume excess?
7. Describe diagnostic testing to monitor fluid status.
8. List various IV solutions and their use.
9. Describe several nursing measures to reduce patients' risk for fluid imbalances.
10. What is the effect of potassium on the body?

## APPLY WHAT YOU LEARNED

A newly admitted 28-year-old female diagnosed with hypokalemia tells the nurse she drinks mostly water and tea and doesn't really eat solid foods. Her treatment plan will involve IV fluids and a nutritional consult. She will also have cardiac testing done.

1. What are some foods the dietician will recommend to this patient?
2. According to the data given here, would the nurse request any other consults?
3. What types of medication would the nurse expect to see ordered?

## MULTIPLE CHOICE

Circle the answer that best completes the following statements.

1. The primary electrolyte that controls the water balance in the body is:
   A. sodium.
   B. potassium.
   C. chloride.
   D. magnesium.

2. Which of the following patients would be considered at greatest risk for dehydration?
   A. Overweight male
   B. Average-weight male
   C. Underweight female
   D. Overweight female

3. Of the following, which is not considered a function of an electrolyte?
   A. Regulate acid–base balance
   B. Maintain good nutrition
   C. Maintain neuromuscular activity
   D. Assist with enzyme reactions

4. Osmosis is the movement of:
   A. particles across a semipermeable membrane.
   B. water from an area of low-solute concentration to an area of higher concentration.
   C. water and solutes across the capillary membranes.
   D. solutes from an area of low concentration to an area of higher concentration.

5. *Active transport* is defined as:
   A. a sodium–potassium pump.
   B. the movement of molecules from an area of low-solute concentration to an area of high-solute concentration via the ATP mechanism.
   C. cells in a constant state of motion.
   D. molecules that continually move in and out of cells.

6. Mr. Smith has recently been diagnosed with a kidney dysfunction. He constantly complains of thirst. Which of the following statements to the patient BEST indicates the nurse's understanding of the thirst mechanism?

   A. "Thirst is the primary regulator of water intake. When we are thirsty, we drink."

   B. "Thirst is important in maintaining fluid balance and preventing dehydration."

   C. "Thirst mechanisms decline with age, making the older adult at risk for dehydration."

   D. "A drop in blood volume stimulates the thirst center in the brain, which produces the sensation of thirst."

7. The mechanism of action for the antidiuretic hormone (ADH) may be understood as:

   A. kidneys reabsorbing more water when the hormone is present.

   B. kidneys ceasing urine production when the hormone is present.

   C. blood osmolality increasing as urine output decreases.

   D. the hypothalamus detecting increased osmolality of the blood and stimulating the release of ADH.

8. The pathophysiology of SIADH is described as:

   A. the failure of the hypothalamus to release antidiuretic hormone.

   B. an excess of antidiuretic hormone in the bloodstream.

   C. water retention.

   D. copious amounts of concentrated urine.

9. Diabetes insipidus is caused by:

   A. failure of the hypothalamus to release antidiuretic hormone, resulting in excessive amounts of dilute urine.

   B. failure of the hypothalamus to release antidiuretic hormone, resulting in concentrated urine.

   C. failure of the pancreas to produce insulin, resulting in polyuria.

   D. total absence of antidiuretic hormone, resulting in severe water retention.

10. Alice is a 2-year-old child who has been suffering from vomiting and diarrhea for 3 days. Her temperature is 102°F, and she appears lethargic and exhausted. Her mother reports that Alice has not been able to keep anything down. Based on this information, Alice's primary nursing diagnosis should be:

    A. Activity Intolerance.

    B. Deficient Fluid Volume.

    C. Altered Nutrition: Less Than Body Requirements.

    D. Risk for Diarrhea.

11. Your patient has been admitted for uncontrollable vomiting. The doctor has ordered a Foley catheter and an IV of $D_5$ 1/2 NS at 75 mL/hr. After the Foley was inserted, the initial amount of urine obtained was 100 mL. The IV was successfully begun, but 1 hour later the patient's Foley bag had drained only 50 mL. Your next action would be to:

    A. administer an antiemetic in an attempt to stop the loss of gastric fluid.

    B. call the physician and report the low urine output.

    C. continue to monitor.

    D. encourage the patient to increase PO fluids.

12. Which electrolyte is most readily excreted by the kidneys and will be lost even when other electrolytes are conserved?

    A. Potassium

    B. Sodium

    C. Magnesium

    D. Calcium

13. Which of the following statements is FALSE regarding the acid–base balance system?

    A. Blood buffers react quickly but are limited.

    B. The respiratory system adjusts the acid–base balance by either slowing or increasing respirations.

    C. The renal system is the slowest of the systems but is responsible for long-term balance.

    D. When hydrogen ions and the pH in the blood increase, the result is acidosis.

14. A patient suffering from metabolic acidosis is most likely to:

    A. experience an increase in the blood pH.

    B. develop tachypnea.

    C. recover slowly, due to the kidney's role in acid–base balance.

    D. be diagnosed with acute pneumonia.

15. Mr. Jacobs, who was diagnosed with COPD 5 years ago, has been using his oxygen at home via nasal cannula. The flow rate is set at 2 L/min. Mr. Jacobs's respirations are 28/min, and he complains of SOB after minimal exertion. His wife is concerned that the amount of oxygen is "too low." Your best response should be:

    A. "I can't change the flow rate without an order."

    B. "Okay, let's increase the flow rate to 6 L/min and see how he does."

    C. "Increasing his oxygen may actually inhibit the respiratory center in his brain."

    D. "I'll call the doctor and let him know about your concerns."

# CHAPTER 8 ▶ *Caring for Patients in Pain*

## KEY TERMS

Match each term with its appropriate definition.

1. Pain
2. Analgesics
3. Acute pain
4. Opioids
5. Pain threshold
6. Chronic pain
7. PCA
8. Addiction
9. Pain tolerance
10. Opioid tolerance

A. Drugs that can be given alone for moderate to severe pain

B. Seeking drugs for nonmedical reasons

C. Amount of pain endured before seeking relief

D. Patient-controlled analgesia; allows patients to manage pain

E. Unpleasant sensory or emotional experience

F. Usually temporary, has a sudden onset, and is localized

G. Loss of opioid effectiveness with chronic use

H. Processing of pain impulses in the brain

I. Prolonged, persists after the condition causing it has resolved, and may not be an identifiable cause

J. Used to relieve or reduce pain

## LEARNING OUTCOMES

1. What is the difference between pain tolerance and pain threshold?
2. Contrast acute pain and chronic pain.
3. List several factors that affect patient response to pain.
4. What is patient-controlled analgesia?
5. What subjective data might be gathered when assessing a patient's pain?
6. What objective data may be seen in patients with pain?
7. What are some misconceptions about pain management?
8. List several nursing interventions for chronic pain.
9. Name several methods of complementary therapy.
10. What are possible side effects of opioid analgesics?

## APPLY WHAT YOU LEARNED

A 37-year-old patient is seen at a follow-up for chronic back pain. She rates her pain as 7 on a 0–10 scale, and she is out of medication. She was given a prescription for a 30-day supply 2 weeks ago. She then tells the nurse she has been laid off from her job, and her rent is late.

1. How would the nurse question the patient about being out of medication?
2. What subjective and objective findings would the nurse expect to find in this patient with a pain rating of 7?
3. What nonpharmacological interventions could the nurse give this patient?
4. Should the nurse be concerned with addiction? Why or why not?

## MULTIPLE CHOICE

Circle the answer that best completes the following statements.

1. Natalie, a 26-year-old college student, has been admitted to your unit for observation. Recently she has frequently been found crying alone in her room. She admits that she is constantly tired and irritable. The medical history reveals that Natalie was injured in a motor vehicle crash 2 years ago and that she has never fully recovered. Natalie states that her back never stops hurting. You suspect that this may be diagnosed as:
   A. chronic malignant pain.
   B. acute pain syndrome.
   C. chronic nonmalignant pain.
   D. psychosomatic pain.

2. The nurse is caring for a patient who received multiple fractures and contusions from a fall 5 days ago. At 3:30 P.M., the nurse administers the pain medication that was ordered q.i.d. At 5:00 P.M., the patient calls for more pain medication. The assessment shows a BP of 160/88 and a pulse of 100. The nurse checks the chart and discovers that the patient made constant requests for pain relief on the previous shift. The best response would be to:
   A. ignore the patient, as it appears he may be addicted to the medication.
   B. call the physician and report the addiction.
   C. administer another dose at 7:00 P.M.
   D. notify the physician that the current medication may not be effective.

3. Mrs. Hamrick is recovering from knee replacement surgery. Her pain medication order reads as follows: Vicodin 5/500 mg tabs 2 PO q.i.d. PRN pain. She is scheduled for physical therapy from 10:00 to 11:00 A.M. It is now 7:00 A.M. She has not received a tab since 3:00 A.M. You will expect to administer the medication:
   A. at 9:30 A.M.
   B. at 10:00 A.M.
   C. after she returns from therapy.
   D. as soon as she calls for the medication.

4. Timothy, a 10-year-old, has twisted his ankle playing baseball. His mom asks you what other methods could be used to control the pain if the ordered medication does not work. You suggest:

   A. bringing Timothy back to the clinic.

   B. having him read his favorite joke book.

   C. doubling the medication dosage.

   D. placing warm packs on the ankle continuously for 24 hours.

5. A 70-year-old patient with a history of Parkinson disease and arthritis has been placed on Darvocet N100 1 tab PO t.i.d. PRN pain. Which of the following would be a priority nursing diagnosis?

   A. Constipation

   B. Disturbed Thought Processes

   C. Risk for Injury

   D. Activity Intolerance

6. Your patient requires discharge teaching regarding his pain medication, Demerol tabs. Which of the following would be considered your highest priority teaching?

   A. Do not take the medication with alcohol.

   B. Constipation may occur.

   C. Sleepiness is a common side effect.

   D. Nausea can be decreased by taking the medication with food.

7. Mrs. Johnnie has been ordered a PCA pump for pain control after her colon surgery. She voices concern about the potential for overdosing. Your best reply would be:

   A. "Don't worry, that never happens."

   B. "The pump is preset, and you will be allowed to receive only that amount."

   C. "I'll teach you to use the pump and regulate the amount that you get."

   D. "If you are worried about it, we can give you injections instead."

8. A patient has been receiving a new pain medication every 4 hours as ordered. His wife is concerned that he is very sleepy all the time and may be overmedicated. Your best response would be:

   A. "It really is strange that he is that sleepy."

   B. "I'll call the doctor. Thanks for telling me."

   C. "It is not unexpected with a new pain medication. We are checking him every 2 hours."

   D. "If he doesn't wake up in 4 hours, we'll get the medication changed."

9. You receive a call from a patient who has been on long-term pain medications. She is worried that the pharmacist gave her "cheap stuff" because it does not help her pain. The patient may be developing:

   A. increased pain.

   B. tolerance to the medication.

   C. decreased pain tolerance.

   D. chronic pain.

10. Mrs. Wesley is at the doctor's office for a checkup. She asks you why the doctor would prescribe an antidepressant when she is complaining of pain. She says, "I'm not crazy, my back has just hurt for so long." You base your response on the fact that:

    A. antidepressants are capable of relieving many types of pain.

    B. pain can cause confusion.

    C. chronic pain can affect mood and sleep patterns.

    D. opioids work best when taken with other medications.

11. A 17-year-old boy was admitted to the emergency department for fractures received during a football game. He is moaning and crying. After watching you administer a shot of Demerol, the father asks, "Why is my son acting like a baby? He's never acted like this before when a bone was broken!" Your response is based on the fact that:

    A. everyone perceives pain differently.

    B. everyone has a different pain threshold.

    C. previous experiences with pain can affect future coping behaviors.

    D. all of the above.

12. The tool used to measure pain is called a:

    A. pain tolerance guide.

    B. pain threshold scale.

    C. pain conduction tool.

    D. pain scale.

13. Increased blood pressure, dilated pupils, perspiration, and pallor are signs of:

    A. opiate overdose.

    B. acute pain.

    C. adverse effects of Demerol.

    D. chronic pain.

14. Chronic nonmalignant pain is:

    A. known as cancer pain.

    B. due to back pain.

    C. ongoing pain caused by non-life-threatening causes.

    D. ongoing pain caused by a malignant tumor.

15. Response to pain is affected by:

    A. family and cultural expectations.

    B. pain tolerance.

    C. past experiences with pain.

    D. all of the above.

# CHAPTER 9

# Caring for Patients With Inflammation and Infection

## KEY TERMS

Match each term with its appropriate definition.

1. Macrophages
2. Phagocytosis
3. Lymphadenopathy
4. Leukocytosis
5. Abscesses
6. Standard Precautions
7. Infectious disease
8. Antibiotics
9. Pathogens
10. Endogenous pyrogens

A. Guidelines for the handling of blood and other body fluids to protect the health care worker and prevent transmission to other patients

B. Enlargement of the lymph nodes as a systemic response to inflammation

C. Chemicals released by macrophages that cause fever

D. Medications used to treat bacterial infection

E. Illness that results from infection

F. Large WBCs that ingest harmful bacteria and dead tissue

G. Pockets in which pus develops and accumulates

H. Increased WBC production

I. Process in which neutrophils and macrophages ingest harmful bacteria and dead tissue

J. Microorganisms that are capable of causing disease

## LEARNING OUTCOMES

1. List several factors that would cause inflammation.
2. What are the steps in the inflammatory response?
3. What are the manifestations of local inflammation?
4. What manifestations are associated with systemic inflammation?
5. Name the links in the chain of infection.
6. List several common infectious diseases.
7. What are the risk factors for health care–associated (nosocomial) infections?
8. Identify several Standard Precaution guidelines.
9. What subjective data would be presented by a patient with an infection?
10. What would objective data be in a patient with an infection?

## APPLY WHAT YOU LEARNED

You are caring for a resident recently admitted from a nursing home with a fever and urinary tract infection. The resident has an indwelling Foley catheter. The resident is confused and does not answer questions appropriately. You notice a skin tear on the lower extremity that has no dressing.

1. What lab tests is the nurse expecting to see ordered by the physician?
2. Can the nurse obtain subjective data from this patient? Why or why not?
3. What course of treatment would the nurse expect to be ordered?

## MULTIPLE CHOICE

Circle the answer that best completes the following statements.

1. Edema to an injured or infected site is which step in the inflammatory response?
   A. Vascular
   B. Cellular
   C. Healing
   D. Chemical

2. Nursing interventions for a patient with acute inflammation are aimed at which cardinal manifestations of inflammation?
   A. Redness, swelling, pain
   B. Warmth, pain, impaired function
   C. Swelling, impaired function, pain
   D. Redness, warmth, impaired function

3. You examine a WBC count ordered for a patient. The WBC count is 3,000/mm³. This value most likely indicates:
   A. leukocytosis, a bacterial infection.
   B. leukopenia, a viral infection.
   C. a normal WBC count.
   D. no information of value.

4. When interpreting a WBC differential, a "shift to the left" indicates which of the following?
   A. Large number of immature WBCs, severe infection
   B. Large number of mature WBCs, severe infection
   C. Large number of immature WBCs, cancer
   D. Large number of mature WBCs, cancer

5. Cultures of blood, wounds, or other infected body fluids should be obtained:
   A. 30 minutes after the first dose of antimicrobial therapy.
   B. 24 hours after the first dose of antimicrobial therapy.
   C. 24 and 36 hours after the first dose of antimicrobial therapy.
   D. prior to beginning antimicrobial therapy.

6. The nurse wears personal protective equipment (gloves, mask, gown, and goggles) to break which link in the chain of infection?
   A. Microorganism
   B. Reservoir
   C. Portal of exit
   D. Portal of entry

7. Choose the nursing intervention that will break the chain of infection in a patient with a contagious respiratory infection.
   A. Administer antibiotic therapy.
   B. Have all visitors wear a mask.
   C. Practice meticulous hand washing.
   D. All of the above.

8. Which of the following microorganisms is easily transmitted from patient to patient via a nurse's hands?
   A. *Escherichia coli*
   B. *Staphylococcus aureus*
   C. Streptococci
   D. Enterococcus

9. Inappropriate use of antibiotics contributes to health care–associated (nosocomial) infections because:
   A. some bacteria survive and become resistant to the antibiotic.
   B. normal flora are killed.
   C. infections occur only in those people who are taking antibiotics.
   D. none of the above.

10. You are changing linens for a patient with a draining wound infected with MRSA. Which precautions should be taken?
    A. Wear gloves, gown, and mask to change linens.
    B. Wear gloves to change linens.
    C. Wear gloves and gown to change linens.
    D. No precautions are necessary.

11. Which of the following patients is at greatest risk for infection?
    A. 42-year-old patient with a rib fracture
    B. 56-year-old patient with enlarged prostate who drinks cranberry juice
    C. 62-year-old patient with a history of TB exposure
    D. 76-year-old patient with a recent CVA and no flu vaccine

12. Penicillin should be taken:
    A. with food.
    B. with yogurt.
    C. with water.
    D. until symptoms dissipate.

13. An example of a cephalosporin is:

    A. cefazolin.

    B. nafcillin.

    C. potassium clavulanate.

    D. gentamycin.

14. The CDC recommends what as the preferred method of hand hygiene?

    A. Wearing gloves and changing them frequently

    B. Using an alcohol-based hand rub

    C. Using nonantiseptic soaps

    D. None of the above

15. You are caring for a hospitalized patient who develops chickenpox after a visit from his 5-year-old son. Your patient will require which level of precaution?

    A. Negative air pressure room with visitors wearing a mask

    B. Private room with visitors wearing a mask within 3 ft

    C. Gown and gloves required if entering room

    D. No precautions other than standard

# CHAPTER 10 ▸ *Caring for Patients Having Surgery*

## KEY TERMS

Match each term with its appropriate definition.

1. Shock
2. Drain
3. Postoperative phase
4. Emancipated minors
5. Dehiscence
6. Informed consent
7. Secondary intention
8. Ambulatory surgery
9. Intraoperative phase
10. Evisceration

A. Period beginning with entry into the operating room

B. Surgical procedure performed in a physician's office, free-standing surgery center, or hospital facility

C. Operative permit

D. Protrusion of body organs from a wound

E. Life-threatening postoperative complication that results from insufficient blood flow to vital organs

F. Healing of a large, gaping, irregular wound

G. Separation of incisional wound

H. Person under age 18, lives independently

I. Period beginning with admittance to recovery area

J. Device that promotes the drainage of wound debris and healing from the inside to the outside

## LEARNING OUTCOMES

1. Contrast inpatient surgery and ambulatory surgery.
2. List several important things a perioperative nurse must understand.
3. What are the components of informed consent?
4. List and describe three phases of the surgical experience.
5. What is the focus of preoperative care?
6. Describe nursing care on the day of surgery.
7. What happens in the body under anesthesia?
8. List five hospital national patient safety goals.
9. What is the difference between dehiscence and evisceration?
10. Discuss pain management for the postoperative patient.

## APPLY WHAT YOU LEARNED

You are caring for a postoperative patient with a PCA for pain control. The patient states she is not going to use it due to the fear of addiction. She states that if the pain gets bad enough, she will ring for the nurse.

1. How would the nurse educate the patient regarding the PCA pump?
2. Explain pain control in the postoperative patient.
3. How would the nurse assess the patient's readiness to use the PCA?

## MULTIPLE CHOICE

Circle the answer that best completes the following statements.

1. The nurse should know that the patient's surgery will be postponed if the hemoglobin level is below:
   A. 16 g per 100 mL.
   B. 10 g per 100 mL.
   C. 12 g per 100 mL.
   D. 14 g per 100 mL.

2. A patient with diabetes is more at risk for postoperative complications because:
   A. the prescribed diet cannot be consumed due to nausea.
   B. healing rarely takes place in the diabetic patient.
   C. blood glucose levels can fluctuate uncontrollably.
   D. the patient is unable to administer self-injections of insulin.

3. Preoperative medications must be administered:
   A. within 15 minutes of the ordered time.
   B. within 30 minutes of the ordered time.
   C. at the ordered time.
   D. after the skin scrub is completed.

4. While the surgical patient is semiconscious and receiving IV therapy, the nurse should:
   A. keep the arms unrestrained so that the joints will not stiffen.
   B. elevate the arm above the level of the heart.
   C. gently massage the arm to relieve muscle spasms and prevent clots from forming.
   D. monitor the IV site at frequent intervals.

5. Immediately following surgery, the patient's vital signs must be checked every:
   A. 5 minutes.
   B. 15 minutes.
   C. 20 minutes.
   D. 30 minutes.

6. Your patient calls you to his room and tells you that something is wrong with his incision. You notice that the edges of the wound have separated and a small amount of beefy red tissue is observable. Your first response should be to:

   A. notify the physician.

   B. cover the wound with sterile dry dressing.

   C. place a sterile dressing moistened with normal saline over the wound.

   D. ask the patient how long ago this occurred.

7. The nurse will instruct the patient receiving a local anesthetic that:

   A. no pain will be felt during the procedure.

   B. drowsiness is a side effect of the medication.

   C. bleeding is usually superficial.

   D. consciousness will be lost.

8. The nurse should teach the patient that, after surgery, DVT may be prevented by:

   A. raising the head of the bed.

   B. engaging in passive and active leg exercises.

   C. keeping the knees elevated.

   D. encouraging coughing and deep-breathing exercises.

9. Which of the following patients is at a greater risk for developing postsurgical and postanesthesia complications?

   A. 42-year-old scheduled for eye surgery

   B. 3-year-old scheduled for a hernia repair

   C. 80-year-old scheduled for a right hip replacement

   D. 18-year-old scheduled for a cervical biopsy

10. You are asked to obtain an informed consent for a patient who is scheduled for a bowel resection. Your main responsibility should be to:

    A. explain the risks involved with the surgery.

    B. discuss other medical options that might be useful for this patient's condition.

    C. witness the patient's signature of consent.

    D. check the form for completeness.

11. Your patient is scheduled for surgery in 2 hours. He asks you why the surgery has to be done right away. He insists on a detailed explanation of the procedure. The legal responsibility for explaining the procedure rests with the:

    A. charge nurse.

    B. hospital risk management team.

    C. physician who will perform the surgery.

    D. patient advocate.

12. Coughing and deep breathing are techniques that must be taught to surgical patients to prevent:

    **A.** the formation of clots at the incision site.

    **B.** lung collapse after the surgery.

    **C.** hypotension.

    **D.** prolonged pain.

13. Morphine and Fentanyl may be ordered as a preoperative medication to:

    **A.** eliminate spasms of the colon.

    **B.** enhance the effects of the anesthetic.

    **C.** decrease hypertensive episodes during surgery.

    **D.** reduce pain while in the recovery room.

14. It is important for the nurse to assess the patient's home medications prior to surgery because:

    **A.** these medications may alter the patient's perception of the surgery.

    **B.** the anesthetics received in the operative phase may cause toxicity of other drugs.

    **C.** some medications may interact with the anesthetics, causing undesired effects.

    **D.** routine medications are usually withheld the day of the surgery.

15. Mr. James is complaining of abdominal discomfort 2 days after his hernia repair. He tells you that he feels bloated and has no appetite. Your next action should be to:

    **A.** tell the patient that this is normal and to ambulate as much as possible.

    **B.** ask Mr. James about his last bowel movement.

    **C.** assess bowel function.

    **D.** administer a stool softener.

# CHAPTER 11 ▶ Caring for Patients With Altered Immunity

## KEY TERMS

Match each term with its appropriate definition.

1. Antigen
2. Desensitization
3. Helper T cells
4. Seroconversion
5. AIDS
6. Human papillomavirus
7. Toxoid
8. Memory cells
9. Hypersensitivity
10. Immunocompetent

A. Produce specific antibody when reexposed to a specific antigen
B. Responsible for switching on the immune system
C. Virus causing genital warts
D. Final, fatal stage of HIV infection
E. Any nonself substance
F. Process in which B-cell antibodies are produced
G. Form of immunotherapy that involves injecting small doses of the allergen weekly
H. Person whose immune system identifies and effectively destroys antigens
I. Substances that contain an inactivated toxin that is produced by a microbe
J. Altered immune response in which the body overreacts to an antigen

## LEARNING OUTCOMES

1. What is the function of a leukocyte?
2. Identify the cells of the immune system.
3. What are the differences between IgG and IgA?
4. Contrast active and passive immunity.
5. List several recommended immunizations for adults.
6. What is anaphylaxis?
7. Describe the four types of hypersensitivity reactions.
8. Name several natural rubber latex products.
9. What are autoimmune disorders?
10. List several manifestations of HIV infection.

## APPLY WHAT YOU LEARNED

You are caring for a patient who is newly diagnosed with HIV. There has been a positive diagnosis of Kaposi sarcoma, and on visualization, there are white patches in the mouth. The patient is a 28-year-old male, and his partner is at the bedside trying to comfort him and help him relax.

1. How would the nurse explain Kaposi sarcoma to the patient and his partner?
2. What are the white patches in the mouth of this patient?
3. What nursing interventions can be implemented to assist the patient and his partner regarding relaxation?

## MULTIPLE CHOICE

Circle the answer that best completes the following statements.

1. The function of the bone marrow is to:
   A. mature lymphocytes into T cells.
   B. filter out damaged RBCs.
   C. manufacture blood cells.
   D. filter out foreign particles.

2. A nursing assistant tells the nurse that a rash is developing on her hands. The most appropriate response should be:
   A. "What are you washing your hands with?"
   B. "Don't wear any gloves when you give a bath."
   C. "Which type of gloves are you using?"
   D. "Do you have an allergy to peanuts?"

3. The nurse is providing teaching for a patient scheduled for allergy skin testing. The patient asks what kind of preparation is needed for the test. The best response might be:
   A. "You don't need to do anything."
   B. "Oh, I have to gather all the supplies for the doctor."
   C. "Nothing, but epinephrine will be given prior to the test."
   D. None of the above.

4. Adults should have a tetanus toxoid (Td) every:
   A. year.
   B. 2 years.
   C. 5 years.
   D. 10 years.

5. The nurse is teaching a "safe-sex" class at a local high school. He knows that further teaching is necessary when one of the students states:
   A. "As long as I use a condom, I won't get anyone pregnant."
   B. "Wow, I didn't know that condoms should be made of latex."
   C. "I shouldn't have unprotected sex."
   D. "I guess that the condoms in my wallet are too old to use now."

6. You are assessing a patient's immune status. Which of the following must be included in the documentation?
   A. Recent exposure to a friend with active tuberculosis
   B. Hernia repair 4 years ago
   C. Diagnosis of posttraumatic stress syndrome
   D. Low-pitched bowel sounds

7. You are preparing for the NCLEX-PN® by reviewing your immunology notes. Which of the following is NOT considered a part of the immune system?
   A. Thymus gland
   B. Appendix
   C. Gallbladder
   D. Spleen

8. A patient has been taking diphenhydramine for hay fever symptoms. Which of the following is NOT a common side effect of the medication?
   A. Drowsiness
   B. Sedation
   C. Urinary retention
   D. Thirst

9. A patient is taking cyclosporine to prevent the rejection of his new kidney. The daily lab work is faxed to your unit. Which of the following would require a call to the physician?
   A. Glucose 93
   B. BUN 10
   C. WBC 3,000
   D. Platelet count 150,000

10. You feel confident that your patient, an organ transplant recipient, understands your discharge instructions when he says:
    A. "I'm going to take my temperature and weight at the same time every day."
    B. "Since I will be taking CellCept, I will be sure to drink more water than usual."
    C. "As long as I don't drink from the same glass after my children when they are sick, I will be safe from infection."
    D. "I won't have to see my doctor unless I don't feel well."

11. Nursing care for any immunocompromised patient includes removing invasive lines as soon as possible. The rationale for this intervention is that:
    A. the patient can go home sooner.
    B. fewer sites are available for bacterial invasion.
    C. the patient is more comfortable.
    D. signs of infection are easier to monitor.

12. Isolation Precautions for the transplant patient are designed to:
    A. reduce possible microorganisms transferred by the patient.
    B. reduce possible microorganisms transferred to the patient.
    C. reduce the risk of rejection.
    D. all of the above.

13. Your patient, a 62-year-old female, has recently been diagnosed with rheumatoid arthritis. She tells you that she just doesn't feel like getting up in the mornings. Her housework is not getting done. An appropriate nursing diagnosis might be:

   A. Disturbed Body Image.

   B. Fatigue.

   C. Ineffective Individual Coping.

   D. Acute Pain.

14. In addition to the ELISA, which of the following tests is used to diagnose HIV?

   A. HIV viral load

   B. CD4+ cell count

   C. Western blot

   D. All of the above

15. The appropriate statement to a patient who admitted to "sharing a needle" should be:

   A. "If your HIV test is negative after 3 months, you have nothing to fear."

   B. "Don't worry, the HIV virus is transmitted only by semen."

   C. "Seroconversion usually occurs in 6 to 24 weeks."

   D. "Try not to think about it."

## KEY TERMS

Match each term with its appropriate definition.

1. Cancer
2. Oncology
3. Neoplasm
4. Metastasis
5. Carcinogenesis
6. Benign
7. Anorexia–cachexia syndrome
8. Biotherapy
9. Carcinogens
10. Malignant

A. Occurs when normal cells mutate into abnormal cells that grow uncontrollable and spread

B. Tumors with localized growths with well-defined borders; tend to respond to the body's controls

C. Process in which normal cells are transformed into cancer cells

D. Study of cancer

E. Uses medications to stimulate the patient's immune system to target and destroy cancer cells

F. Metabolic syndrome associated with cancer

G. Mass of abnormal cells that grows independently of its surrounding structures and has no physiologic purpose

H. Cancer-causing agents

I. Tumors that grow aggressively and do not respond to the body's controls

J. Secondary tumors and the process by which malignant neoplasms spread

## LEARNING OUTCOMES

1. Contrast benign and malignant neoplasms.
2. What is an oncogene?
3. Name several controllable risk factors associated with cancer.
4. List some carcinogens associated with cancer.
5. What are possible cancer warning signs?
6. List several common general manifestations of cancer.
7. What are some signs of anorexia–cachexia syndrome?
8. Describe the tumor classification system.
9. List several oncologic emergencies.
10. What are some common side effects of chemotherapy?

## APPLY WHAT YOU LEARNED

A 65-year-old male was just admitted to your unit with anorexia related to prostate cancer with metastasis to the lungs. Consults have been ordered for dietary and hospice. His wife is at the bedside trying to engage him in conversation about anything other than cancer. He is staring blankly out of the window.

1. What interventions could the nurse use regarding the anorexia?
2. How would the nurse assist the patient and his wife with his grieving?
3. What role will hospice nurses play in the care of this patient?

## MULTIPLE CHOICE

Circle the answer that best completes the following statements.

1. Nurses are aware that the disease with the second-highest mortality rate in the United States is:
   A. chronic obstructive pulmonary disease.
   B. end-stage renal failure.
   C. cancer.
   D. coronary artery disease.

2. You are teaching a health class at a local retirement center. When discussing the potential for prostate cancer in the older male, you include the following teaching point:
   A. prostate self-examination every week
   B. x-ray of the prostate gland after the age of 65
   C. screening for the presence of PSA
   D. CT scan of the chest to rule out metastasis

3. Mrs. Jackson has been diagnosed with breast cancer and metastasis to the spinal cord. She is paralyzed from the waist down and requires assistance with ADLs. Which of the following nursing diagnoses would be the most appropriate at this time?
   A. Risk for Infection
   B. Risk for Impaired Skin Integrity
   C. Risk for Injury
   D. Risk for Caregiver Role Strain

4. A divorced mother of four school-aged children is hospitalized with inoperable brain cancer. The patient voices concern over the care for her children after her death. The best response is:
   A. "You are going to live for a while longer and will have time to make arrangements."
   B. "Won't your ex-husband care for his kids after your death?"
   C. "I wouldn't worry about that right now. Just focus on getting well."
   D. "Would you like to share your thoughts with me?"

5. Interleukin-2 is used as therapy for a patient with metastatic renal cancer. The nurse recognizes that the goal of this type of treatment might be:

   A. selectively altering the DNA of malignant cells.

   B. enhancing the patient's immunologic response to tumor cells.

   C. stimulating malignant cells to enter mitosis.

   D. preventing bone marrow depression.

6. After the implantation of a radioactive cervical implant in an outpatient clinic, it is important to teach the patient to:

   A. avoid close contact with others.

   B. limit activity to 30 minutes per day.

   C. eat three nutritious meals every day.

   D. dispose of the implant in the trash if it becomes dislodged.

7. You are reviewing a patient's history prior to assisting in the development of a nursing care plan. You note that the patient has been diagnosed with colon carcinoma. The staging classification is $T_{IS}$. You understand that this represents:

   A. a tumor with no metastasis.

   B. no evidence of a primary tumor.

   C. a tumor that is localized and encapsulated.

   D. two abnormal lymph nodes.

8. Several cancer warning signals have been identified. If all of the following are true, which signal would be particularly important to the chronic smoker?

   A. Obvious change in mole or wart

   B. A sore that does not heal

   C. Nagging cough

   D. Change in bowel habit

9. The nurse has completed a physical assessment on a patient diagnosed with pancreatic cancer. Which of these findings indicates poor nutritional status?

   A. Positive muscle tone

   B. Good skin turgor

   C. Moist oral membranes

   D. Distended abdomen

10. A gastric cancer patient is receiving high doses of 5-FU. Based on your knowledge of the side effects of this chemotherapy drug, which nursing intervention should take priority in the patient's care?

    A. Six small meals a day

    B. Increase PO fluids

    C. Assess lungs for coarse rales

    D. Monitor lab values for the presence of uric acid

11. The drug tamoxifen is generally used in the treatment of:

    A. breast cancer.

    B. prostate cancer.

    C. small-cell lung cancer.

    D. bladder cancer.

12. A patient who is being treated on an outpatient basis for kidney cancer telephones the nurse on duty and states, "I just don't think I can take any more treatments." The best response of the nurse should be:

    A. "Okay, I'll let your doctor know right away."

    B. "You sound terrible, what's the matter?"

    C. "Would you like to talk about your concerns?"

    D. "Please tell me your concerns."

13. Which of the following are NOT characteristics of a malignant neoplasm?

    A. Rapid growth

    B. Well-defined borders

    C. Noncohesive

    D. Invasive

14. The nurse is teaching the patient about the care of radiation skin markings. Of the following, which should be most emphasized during the session?

    A. Protect the skin from sunlight.

    B. Do not wash off the markings.

    C. Do not apply heat or cold to the marked areas.

    D. Wear loose clothing.

15. The nurse understands that which of the following is NOT a common psychologic response to a diagnosis of cancer?

    A. Guilt

    B. Hypoglycemia

    C. Fear

    D. Anger

# CHAPTER 13 ▶ *Loss, Grief, and End-of-Life Care*

## KEY TERMS

Match each term with its appropriate definition.

1. Loss
2. Grief
3. Death
4. Advance directives
5. Durable power of attorney for health care
6. Living will
7. Comfort measures only order
8. Euthanasia
9. Hospice
10. DNR order

A. Irreversible cessation of brain function

B. Personal expression of desires for end-of-life interventions

C. Planning for health care/financial matters in the event of incapacitation

D. Order indicating no life-sustaining measures; providing only soothing interventions at end of life

E. Emotional response to loss

F. Killing that is prompted by some humanitarian motive

G. Transfer of power to another person for decisions in care

H. Absence or potential absence of a valued object, person, body part, or situation that was normally present

I. Model for end-of-life care in the face of limited life expectancy

J. Order written by the physician stating the patient is not to be resuscitated in the case of respiratory or cardiac arrest

## LEARNING OUTCOMES

1. Define *palliative care*.
2. What are Kübler-Ross's stages of grief?
3. List several common fears related to loss.
4. Describe the three types of advance directives.
5. What is the difference between a do-not-resuscitate order and a comfort measures only order?
6. List several ways the nurse can support the dying patient and her family.
7. List several manifestations of impending death.
8. Identify comfort measures for the patient nearing death.
9. What is the role of hospice?
10. Describe the physiologic changes that indicate death.

## APPLY WHAT YOU LEARNED

The nurse arrives to work at the hospice unit to find that there is a new admission. The patient is an 84-year-old male with end-stage Alzheimer disease. The patient's daughter, son, and grandson are present for the admission. The patient is unaware of his current surroundings and appears to be pleasant.

1. How would the nurse describe to the family members the type of care the patient is going to receive?
2. How would the nurse explain nursing procedures to the patient?
3. Explain the process of impending death as the nurse would describe it to the family.

## MULTIPLE CHOICE

Circle the answer that best completes the following statements.

1. A nursing student tells the nurse that she has heard the "death rattle" while caring for a patient. The best explanation of this term is:
    A. creaking of the joints.
    B. gurgling of fluids in the lungs and throat.
    C. air bubbles in the stomach.
    D. teeth grinding.

2. Factors that may interfere with successful grieving include all of the following EXCEPT:
    A. traumatic circumstances surrounding the loss.
    B. perceived inability to share the loss.
    C. lack of social recognition of the loss.
    D. mutual understanding and relationships.

3. The process of viewing the body after death best supports which of the following statements?
    A. Provides resolution of the death experience for most families
    B. Increases anxiety levels
    C. Allows family members an avenue of escape from the truth
    D. Supports the family members' decision for a DNR

4. Which of the following would most likely interfere with the nurse–patient relationship during the final stages of impending death?
    A. Unresolved issues of the nurse's perception of death
    B. Anger with the physician for writing a DNR order
    C. Inability to notify the patient's family of the impending death
    D. Personal knowledge of the patient's family situation

5. A nurse is caring for an older Chinese American patient and notices that a piece of handkerchief is lying on her chest. As soon as possible, the nurse should:
    A. throw the cloth in the trash.
    B. place the item on the bedside table.
    C. speak to the family about the significance of the gesture.
    D. ignore the distraction.

6. An American Indian family appears to be throwing a party in the room where their grandmother is dying. Your best response would be to:
   A. remind the family of the seriousness of the situation.
   B. join in the festivities.
   C. acknowledge the cultural tradition.
   D. report the incident to the nursing supervisor.

7. A nursing assistant refuses to care for a dying person. The most appropriate response by the nurse would be:
   A. "Okay, I'll reassign you to another patient."
   B. "Please tell me what concerns you about this patient's care."
   C. "Grow up—death is a part of life!"
   D. "Just get someone else to do this assignment for you."

8. Physical and emotional care is important to the dying person. Which of the following interventions would be the most comforting during the last stages of life?
   A. Change the linens every 2 hours.
   B. Provide frequent oral care.
   C. Encourage a family member to spend time at the bedside.
   D. Tell the patient that everything will be okay.

9. The concern that most patients voice as they near the end of their lives is the fear of:
   A. dying alone.
   B. pain.
   C. leaving family members.
   D. bodily function loss.

10. You are helping another nurse turn a comatose, dying patient. The nurse states, "Whew! This lady sure is fat." Your best response would be:
    A. "That's not a nice thing to say."
    B. "Yeah, you got that right!"
    C. "Let's talk outside after we are finished."
    D. Say nothing; just glare at the nurse.

11. A 94-year-old patient refuses to eat breakfast. According to the shift report, she has not eaten in 3 days. Your next action should be to:
    A. keep trying to feed her by placing the food in her mouth.
    B. read the physician's notes in her chart.
    C. call the family and ask them to bring food from home.
    D. start an IV of $D_5W$ to provide calories.

12. Your patient, diagnosed with inoperable stomach cancer, wants to die at home. He asks you what organization might help him die peacefully. Which of the following would be the most appropriate community referral resource?
    A. Meals on Wheels
    B. Community mental health centers
    C. Hospice
    D. American Association of Colleges of Nursing

13. The nurse is aware that a terminal patient has stopped breathing and responds to the call only after drinking a cup of coffee. This type of behavior is considered:

    A. routine in most facilities.

    B. malpractice if the patient has not been designated a DNR.

    C. unprofessional and inhumane.

    D. appropriate considering the patient's prognosis.

14. You are caring for a patient with end-stage renal disease. The patient is fully alert and competent. The husband asks, "Give my wife just a little more pain medication to completely stop her from suffering." Your best response would be to:

    A. clarify the request.

    B. privately administer more medication.

    C. speak to the wife about her pain level.

    D. call the physician and report the incident.

15. You overhear a patient state, "If you make me well, God, I will try to be a better person." You know that this type of statement is one of the stages of the grieving process known as:

    A. anger.

    B. bargaining.

    C. denial.

    D. depression.

# CHAPTER 14

# Caring for Patients Experiencing Shock, Trauma, or Disasters

## KEY TERMS

Match each term with its appropriate definition.

1. Triage
2. ICU psychosis
3. Shock
4. Ischemia
5. Type and cross-match
6. ARDS
7. DIC
8. Septicemia
9. Positive inotropic drugs
10. Vasopressor drug

A. Acute condition characterized by simultaneous bleeding and clotting throughout the body

B. Acute confusion after 2 to 3 days in the ICU

C. Reduced blood supply to an organ

D. Drugs that increase the force of myocardial contraction to increase cardiac output

E. Acute respiratory failure due to damage to the alveoli

F. Drugs that produce vasoconstriction to raise the patient's blood pressure

G. Presence of pathogens and pathogenic toxins in the blood

H. System to identify priority of care

I. Test to determine donor and recipient ABO types and Rh groups

J. Life-threatening condition with inadequate blood flow to tissues and cells

## LEARNING OUTCOMES

1. Name five types of shock.
2. Describe the three stages of shock.
3. What are the common causes for hypovolemic shock?
4. What are manifestations of anaphylactic shock?
5. What is autotransfusion?
6. Identify the four types of blood and blood products.
7. List important nursing implications for blood transfusions.
8. What is trauma?
9. Contrast blunt and penetrating trauma.
10. Identify home safety tips to prevent injuries.

## APPLY WHAT YOU LEARNED

A 22-year-old male enters the emergency department after being hit on the head with a baseball while watching a game. There is no active bleeding, but he is complaining of a headache and some blurred vision. You notice that he is also holding his head where the injury occurred.

1. How would this injury be classified?
2. What assessment questions would the nurse ask during triage?
3. What diagnostic testing and treatments would the nurse expect to see ordered by the physician?

## MULTIPLE CHOICE

Circle the answer that best completes the following statements.

1. Which of the following would NOT be considered the cause of a blood pressure drop in the condition known as shock?
   A. Loss of blood volume
   B. Severe histamine reaction
   C. Decreased cardiac output
   D. Low HGB and HCT

2. A patient with end-stage kidney disease is at risk for the progressive stage of shock because the:
   A. kidneys are not able to concentrate urine.
   B. renin–angiotensin–aldosterone system is not functioning properly.
   C. kidneys are not able to metabolize toxins.
   D. patient is not at risk for this stage of shock.

3. Mr. Jones admits to the emergency department in shock after a motor vehicle crash. He is disoriented and unable to follow simple commands. You know that this is due to:
   A. decreased blood flow to the brain.
   B. vasoconstriction of the great vessels.
   C. shunting of blood to the GI tract.
   D. stress caused by the crash.

4. A person is most likely to experience an anaphylactic reaction:
   A. within 5 minutes of exposure to the allergen.
   B. after the second day of exposure to the allergen.
   C. when exposed to any allergen that produces hypersensitivity.
   D. during the second exposure to the allergen.

5. Mrs. James is recovering from septic shock. She has extensive tissue damage to her liver and kidneys due to:
   A. bacterial infection.
   B. reaction to the antibiotic.
   C. endotoxins released into the bloodstream.
   D. microemboli.

6. The administration of oxygen is an appropriate therapy for all types of shock because:

    A. oxygen eases the respiratory effort.

    B. lack of oxygen is the primary cause of tissue damage.

    C. oxygen is considered a comforting measure.

    D. lack of oxygen increases the risk for mental confusion.

7. A patient with B-negative blood requires an emergency transfusion of whole blood. You know that in order to be compatible, the blood obtained from the lab must be:

    A. O negative or B negative.

    B. O positive or B negative or B positive.

    C. B negative or AB negative.

    D. B positive or B negative.

8. The goal of epinephrine therapy is to:

    A. promote bronchiole dilatation and increase arterial BP.

    B. reverse the histamine effects.

    C. prevent a delayed reaction to an antigen.

    D. prevent a delayed reaction to an antibody.

9. The nurse knows that which of the following diagnostic tests is used to determine shock?

    A. Arterial blood gases

    B. X-ray studies

    C. Blood cultures

    D. None of the above

10. Mr. Bruce has a nursing diagnosis of Ineffective Tissue Perfusion related to cardiopulmonary failure. Your primary nursing intervention will be to:

    A. maintain airway and blood oxygen saturation.

    B. check vital signs every hour.

    C. obtain daily weights.

    D. assess bowel function every shift.

11. A patient has been in the trauma room for 15 hours after experiencing a severe injury to her back. You suspect that the shock of the accident is resolving because:

    A. she stops asking where she is.

    B. her urine output has increased to 40 mL/hr and the pedal pulses are palpable.

    C. oxygen saturation levels have been >94% for the last 60 minutes.

    D. her blood pressure is stable at 100/50.

12. You are pulled to the emergency department to assist with a sudden influx of patients. When you arrive, the charge nurse says to "pick a patient." Who will you see first?

    A. 50-year-old, chest pain, BP 140/80

    B. 26-year-old chronic asthmatic, R 30, $O_2$ saturation 92% room air, BP 120/72

    C. 18-year-old, leg trauma from a motor vehicle crash, controlled hemorrhage, BP 139/80

    D. 42-year-old, fall from roof, slurred speech, BP 80/40, P 160, R 36 shallow

13. The home health nurse is visiting 92-year-old Mr. Smith, who has been diagnosed with Parkinson disease and early macular degeneration. Mr. Smith is at risk for trauma related to weakness and poor eyesight. Which of the following would decrease the fall potential for this patient?

    A. Review the medications with the doctor.

    B. Assist the patient in rearranging the furniture.

    C. Increase the number of lamps in the house.

    D. Encourage him to move into assisted-living housing.

14. Andrea has been diagnosed with an allergy to peanuts. You are providing nutritional education. You know that she needs further teaching when she says:

    A. "I need to ask what type of oil is used to fry the foods."

    B. "I need to read all food labels very carefully."

    C. "If I can't see the nuts, then I can eat the food."

    D. "I need to keep Benadryl with me at all times."

15. The school nurse is providing first-aid training to a group of high school athletes. When she discusses hemorrhaging, she remembers to include:

    A. apply a tourniquet immediately to bleeding limbs.

    B. call for help and then apply a tourniquet.

    C. always move an injured person with the head lower than the feet.

    D. check for immediate danger, call for help, and apply pressure.

# CHAPTER 15

# The Cardiovascular System and Assessment

## KEY TERMS

Match each term with its appropriate definition.

1. Peripheral vascular system
2. Blood pressure
3. ECG
4. Systole
5. Peripheral vascular resistance
6. Diastole
7. Cardiac output
8. Cardiovascular system
9. Stroke volume
10. Contractility

A. Natural ability of the cardiac muscle fibers to shorten during systole

B. Force exerted by blood against the walls of the arteries

C. Force opposing blood flow

D. Volume of blood ejected from the heart with each contraction

E. Heart, blood, and blood vessels

F. When the ventricles are relaxed; ventricular filling occurs at this stage

G. When the ventricles contract, ejecting blood into the pulmonary and systemic circuits

H. Network of blood vessels that carry blood to peripheral tissues and return it to the heart

I. Amount of blood pumped by the ventricles in 1 minute

J. Record of the heart's electrical activity detected by electrodes on the skin

## LEARNING OUTCOMES

1. Describe the heart.
2. Contrast diastole and systole.
3. What are the parts of the peripheral vascular system?
4. Describe an ECG.
5. What is poor contractility?
6. Explain cardiac output.
7. List several components that affect heart rate.
8. Identify components of a lipid profile.
9. What imaging studies are used in cardiac dysfunction?
10. What is the purpose of a cardiac MRI?

## APPLY WHAT YOU LEARNED

A nursing student is learning about disruptions related to the cardiac system. The student knows that a complete physical examination is important to provide proper treatment to the patient. The student also knows that assessments need to be performed in a timely manner, especially in acute situations.

1. Describe the type of assessment to be done on a patient experiencing chest pain.
2. Identify diagnostic testing in cardiac dysfunction.

## MULTIPLE CHOICE

Circle the answer that best completes the following statements.

1. The AV valves close as the ventricles start to contract, producing the first heart sound called:
   A. $S_1$.
   B. $S_2$.
   C. $S_3$.
   D. $S_4$.

2. The heartbeat is controlled by specialized cells within the myocardium known as the:
   A. nervous system.
   B. respiratory system.
   C. conduction system.
   D. cardiac system.

3. The sinoatrial (SA) node usually generates an impulse:
   A. 40 to 60 times per minute.
   B. 50 times per minute.
   C. 60 to 100 times per minute.
   D. 100 times per minute.

4. The action potential and depolarization cause muscle to:
   A. beat.
   B. contract.
   C. twitch.
   D. elevate.

5. Ventricular filling occurs when the ventricles are relaxed during:
   A. systole.
   B. heartbeat.
   C. contraction.
   D. diastole.

6. Arteries, veins, and capillaries are included in the:
   A. cardiac system.
   B. GI system.
   C. peripheral vascular system.
   D. pulmonary system.

7. A noninvasive test that has been shown to be highly indicative of atherosclerosis is called a(n):

   A. ankle-brachial index.

   B. ECG.

   C. femoral-cephalic index.

   D. Holter monitor.

8. Which of these hormones are released by the heart muscle in response to changes in blood volume?

   A. ANP

   B. Estrogen

   C. BMP

   D. Testosterone

9. Stress testing is used to detect asymptomatic coronary heart disease and may cause:

   A. a decrease in the pulse rate.

   B. decreased blood pressure.

   C. an increase in stress.

   D. a cardiac emergency.

10. All of the following affect CO, PVR, and BP EXCEPT:

    A. gender.

    B. age.

    C. physical examination.

    D. emotional state.

11. Which part of the heart receives deoxygenated blood from the veins of the body?

    A. Left atrium

    B. Right atrium

    C. Left ventricle

    D. Right ventricle

12. Which structure is known as the "pacemaker" of the heart?

    A. Sinoatrial node

    B. Bundle of His

    C. Purkinje fibers

    D. Left bundle branch

13. The force that opposes blood flow is known as:

    A. arterial resistance.

    B. peripheral vascular resistance.

    C. ventricular resistance.

    D. regurgitation.

14. Which of the following is NOT a part of a lipid profile?

    A. BNP

    B. HDL

    C. LDL

    D. VLDL

15. The bicuspid valve is also known as the:

   **A.** pulmonary valve.

   **B.** mitral valve.

   **C.** aortic valve.

   **D.** tricuspid valve.

## KEY TERMS

Match each term with its appropriate definition.

1. Cardiac arrest
2. Atherosclerosis
3. Angina pectoris
4. Diaphoresis
5. Cardiac dysrhythmia
6. Acute coronary syndrome
7. Ischemic
8. Acute myocardial infarction
9. Unstable angina
10. Cardiogenic shock

A. Profuse sweating

B. Condition of severe cardiac ischemia

C. Medical emergency requiring immediate intervention with CPR measures

D. Causes cells in an area of cardiac muscle die due to lack of blood and oxygen

E. Angina occurring with increasing frequency, at rest, or unpredictably

F. Without enough blood and oxygen to meet metabolic needs

G. A narrowing of the coronary arteries due to plaque formation

H. Impaired tissue perfusion due to pump failure

I. Episodic chest pain

J. Disturbance or irregularity in the heart's electrical system

## LEARNING OUTCOMES

1. List several risk factors for coronary heart disease.
2. What are the proposed steps that lead to atherosclerosis?
3. Describe manifestations of angina.
4. List several manifestations of an acute myocardial infarction.
5. What are two benign reasons for cardiac dysrhythmias?
6. What is cardioversion?
7. Define *sudden cardiac death*.
8. List medications in the class known as calcium channel blockers.
9. What are premature ventricular contractions?
10. Define *atrial flutter*.

## APPLY WHAT YOU LEARNED

You are admitting a patient for a pacemaker insertion. The patient tells you that he has not eaten anything past midnight and has not smoked any cigarettes in the past 24 hours. The patient's wife and teenage daughter are present and will be providing care for him at home.

1. Identify teaching for the patient and the family.
2. What are nursing diagnoses related to this patient?
3. Following discharge, when should the patient call his physician?

## MULTIPLE CHOICE

Circle the answer that best completes the following statements.

1. The nurse is explaining the purpose of an electrocardiogram to a group of nursing students. The nurse would be correct if she said:
   A. "It allows the doctor to view the inside of the heart."
   B. "It produces a picture of the electrical activity of the heart."
   C. "It is used to increase the diameter of the artery."
   D. "It is a device that temporarily takes over the function of the SA node."

2. If all of the following are true, which assessment data should be the highest priority for the nurse to obtain from the patient with a dysrhythmia?
   A. History of falls
   B. Smoking habits
   C. History of cardiovascular disease
   D. Current medications

3. A patient has received instructions on his new pacemaker. Which of these comments, if made by the patient, indicates a need for further teaching?
   A. "I'll carry my pacemaker card in my wallet."
   B. "If my pulse drops lower than the set rate, I'll take a rest break."
   C. "I will call the doctor if I have any chest pain."
   D. "I should see my doctor on a regular schedule."

4. You are walking in the parking lot at a grocery store when you see a woman lying by her car. Your next action should be to:
   A. call for help.
   B. begin CPR.
   C. ask the woman if she is okay.
   D. check for a pulse.

5. A patient presents to the clinic with complaints of orthopnea and severe pedal edema. He tells the nurse that he is taking Lasix and digoxin for congestive heart failure. The assessment reveals an elevated BP, crackles throughout the lung fields, and 3+ pitting edema. The most appropriate nursing diagnosis would be:

   A. Noncompliance.

   B. Ineffective Cardiac Tissue Perfusion.

   C. Risk for Skin Impairment.

   D. Excess Fluid Volume.

6. Several hours after a patient has returned from a coronary angiography, you notice that the dressing is saturated with blood. Your next action should be to:

   A. call the doctor.

   B. check for a pulse distal to the incision.

   C. reinforce the dressing.

   D. apply pressure to the site.

7. Which of the following would NOT be discussed with a patient scheduled for cardiac surgery?

   A. Coughing and deep-breathing exercises

   B. Special cardiac diet prior to the surgery

   C. Visiting hours after the surgery

   D. Proper use of antiembolic hose

8. A patient asks you if his cholesterol level of 210 is within the normal range. Your response should be:

   A. "It all depends on which level you are talking about, the total or the LDL."

   B. "That is high. It should be under 200."

   C. "You have to ask your doctor about that."

   D. "I'm not sure. Let me go check my lab reference book."

9. A patient is to receive a morning dose of digoxin. Which finding, if present, would indicate that the medication should not be given?

   A. Radial pulse of 80

   B. Apical pulse of 52

   C. Radial pulse of 60

   D. Apical pulse of 62

10. A patient with a history of rheumatic heart disease has been scheduled for a tooth extraction. Which of the following would the nurse anticipate the dentist will prescribe for this patient before the procedure?

    A. Anticoagulant

    B. Antibiotic

    C. Cardiotonic

    D. ACE inhibitor

11. Which of the following drugs is a beta-blocker?
    A. Procan
    B. Quinidine
    C. Inderal
    D. Cardizem

12. Which drug class can also cause dysrhythmias?
    A. Beta-blockers
    B. Calcium channel blockers
    C. Digoxins
    D. All of the above

13. What is the first step in the CPR sequence?
    A. Call for help.
    B. Assess for responsiveness.
    C. Open the airway with head tilt–chin lift.
    D. Provide two rescue breaths.

14. Death will follow the onset of V-fib if not treated in:
    A. 30 seconds.
    B. 4 minutes.
    C. 2 minutes.
    D. 10 minutes.

15. Nitroglycerin tablets are given via which method?
    A. Topical
    B. Transdermal
    C. Sublingual
    D. Rectal

# CHAPTER 17

# Caring for Patients With Cardiac Disorders

## KEY TERMS

Match each term with its appropriate definition.

1. Heart failure
2. Acute pulmonary edema
3. Cardiac reserve
4. Orthopnea
5. Stenosis
6. Paroxysmal nocturnal dyspnea
7. Inotropic
8. Cardiac tamponade
9. Rheumatic fever
10. Endocarditis

A. Occurs when valve leaflets fuse together and are unable to open or close fully

B. Breathing difficulty while lying down

C. Condition in which the patient awakens at night acutely short of breath

D. Inflammation of the endocardium, an infectious process that usually affects patients with underlying heart disease

E. Occurs when a rapid buildup of pericardial fluid does not allow the pericardial sac to stretch; can compress the heart

F. Type of drug that increases the strength of the heart's contractions

G. Ability of the heart to adjust its output to meet the metabolic needs of the body

H. A systemic inflammatory disease caused by an abnormal immune response to infection by group A beta-hemolytic streptococci

I. The inability of the heart to function as a pump to meet the needs of the body

J. Accumulation of fluid in the interstitial spaces and alveoli of the lungs

# LEARNING OUTCOMES

1. What are the classifications for heart failure?
2. Identify teaching points for older adults regarding changes in cardiovascular function.
3. Contrast left-sided and right-sided heart failure.
4. List several ways rheumatic fever affects the heart.
5. List several elements of collaborative care related to rheumatic fever.
6. What are the indications for prophylactic antibiotics to prevent endocarditis?
7. Define *pericarditis*.
8. Identify the types of heart murmurs.
9. What is cardiomyopathy?
10. Describe *mitral valve prolapse*.

# APPLY WHAT YOU LEARNED

Your patient was admitted through the emergency department and is to have valvuloplasty in the morning. He has no family present and did not provide you with contact information of any relatives. He states that he lives alone in a two-story home and has to climb 15 stairs to get to his bedroom.

1. What nursing care would be appropriate for this patient after surgery?
2. What other disciplines would the nurse involve in the treatment of this patient?
3. What education should the nurse provide about activity intolerance?

# MULTIPLE CHOICE

Circle the answer that best completes the following statements.

1. You are instructing a nursing student in correct nursing care for a patient taking furosemide. The most important point that should be made at this time is to:

    A. give the drug 1 hour before meals.

    B. assess the apical pulse before administering this drug.

    C. monitor fluid volume status, BP, intake and output, weight, skin turgor, and edema.

    D. use an infusion pump to administer this drug.

2. A patient has been admitted to the hospital with acute heart failure. Which of the following diets would the nurse expect to see ordered for the patient?

    A. Low-fat, high-protein

    B. High-potassium, low-protein

    C. Low-sodium, high-protein

    D. High-protein, high-sodium

3. Which of the following nursing diagnoses would be most appropriate for the patient with congestive heart failure?

    A. Activity Intolerance

    B. Deficient Knowledge

    C. Pain, Acute

    D. Deficient Fluid Volume

4. A patient with end-stage renal disease has been diagnosed with pericarditis. Which intervention would the nurse expect to include in the nursing care plan?

   A. Assist with a pericardiocentesis.

   B. Administer NSAIDs.

   C. Assess the lung sounds every 8 hours.

   D. Place the bed in low-Fowler's position.

5. A 28-year-old female, pregnant with her second child, arrives in the emergency department with severe SOB and hemoptysis. The physician tells you that the patient's lungs are "wet" and that he is able to detect a diastolic murmur. You suspect that this patient has:

   A. aspiration pneumonia.

   B. pulmonary edema.

   C. right-sided heart failure.

   D. cardiac tamponade.

6. Valvular heart disease interferes with blood flow to and from the heart. The most common cause of this disease is:

   A. pericarditis.

   B. MI.

   C. CHF.

   D. rheumatic fever.

7. Valve disorders affect pressures and blood flow both in front of and behind the affected valve. The two major types of heart valve disorders are:

   A. aspiration and pneumonia.

   B. pulmonic and edema.

   C. stenosis and regurgitation.

   D. cardiac and pulmonic.

8. A 34-year-old female, pregnant with her first child, arrives in the emergency department with severe SOB, fatigue, and palpitations. The physician tells you that she is able to detect a diastolic murmur. You suspect that this patient has:

   A. mitral regurgitation.

   B. mitral stenosis.

   C. right-sided heart failure.

   D. cardiac tamponade.

9. You are assessing your patient and hear a "sea gull–like" murmur at the apex of his heart. You suspect that this patient has:

   A. mitral regurgitation.

   B. mitral stenosis.

   C. right-sided heart failure.

   D. cardiac tamponade.

10. A 56-year-old patient presents with angina, dyspnea, and syncope. His prognosis is grim; many patients get progressively worse and die within 2 years of the onset of symptoms without the definitive treatment of cardiac transplant. You suspect that this patient has:

   **A.** cardiac tamponade.

   **B.** myocarditis.

   **C.** cardiomyopathy.

   **D.** pericarditis.

11. The most common cause of right ventricular failure is:

   **A.** left ventricular failure.

   **B.** right atrial failure.

   **C.** left atrial failure.

   **D.** pulmonary failure.

12. The drug class that increases the strength of the heart's contractions is known as:

   **A.** calcium channel blockers.

   **B.** inotropics.

   **C.** analgesics.

   **D.** beta-blockers.

13. A common side effect of an ACE inhibitor is:

   **A.** runny nose.

   **B.** cough.

   **C.** nausea.

   **D.** tinnitus.

14. Cardiac patients need to weigh themselves daily. They should know that 1 kg is equal to:

   **A.** 2.2 kg.

   **B.** 5 pounds.

   **C.** 2.2 pounds.

   **D.** 2.2 cm.

15. Rheumatic fever is usually caused by:

   **A.** *Staphylococcus*.

   **B.** *Streptococcus*.

   **C.** *Clostridium*.

   **D.** *E. coli*.

# CHAPTER 18 ▶ Caring for Patients With Peripheral Vascular Disorders

## KEY TERMS

Match each term with its appropriate definition.

1. Embolus
2. Venous insufficiency
3. Primary hypertension
4. Aneurysm
5. Bruit
6. Thrombus
7. Hypertension
8. Intermittent claudication
9. Deep venous thrombosis
10. Collateral circulation

A. Type of pain described as a cramping or aching sensation in the arch of the foot or calves of the leg

B. A blood clot that has broken away from the vessel wall and moves

C. Harsh or musical sound caused by turbulent blood flow

D. Occurs when a blood clot forms on the wall of a deep vein; common complication of immobility or surgery

E. High blood pressure with no identified cause

F. Blood clot

G. Blood pressure higher than 140 mm Hg systolic or 90 mm Hg diastolic on three separate readings several weeks apart

H. Growth of small blood vessels to maintain tissue perfusion

I. Abnormal dilation of a blood vessel

J. Stasis of venous blood flow in the lower extremities

## LEARNING OUTCOMES

1. List three changes associated with aging that affect older adults' risk for hypertension.
2. Identify risk factors for hypertension.
3. Describe manifestations of an abdominal aortic aneurysm.
4. Define *Marfan syndrome*.
5. Describe *arteriosclerosis*.
6. Identify complementary therapies in peripheral vascular disease (PVD).
7. Define *Raynaud phenomenon*.
8. Identify the risk factors for venous thrombosis.
9. Define *varicose veins*.
10. Describe manifestations of varicose veins.

# APPLY WHAT YOU LEARNED

A 22-year-old woman presents to the emergency department with complaints of stiffness and decreased sensation in her hands. Upon inspection, you notice that over the course of your discussion, her hands have changed from blue to white in color. The patient tells you that her fingers usually turn red after they are white.

1. What would the nurse suspect the diagnosis to be in this patient?
2. Identify treatments regarding this patient.

# MULTIPLE CHOICE

Circle the answer that best completes the following statements.

1. Mr. Greggs, age 68, is being seen in the clinic for a routine physical. He is of Jewish ancestry. He tells you that he smokes a half-pack of cigarettes per day and enjoys popcorn and sodas as a snack. His weight is 205 pounds. Which of these risk factors is considered unalterable in the prevention of hypertension?

   A. Family history

   B. Smoking

   C. High sodium intake

   D. Obesity

2. The nurse is teaching the assistant how to take a blood pressure. Further teaching is indicated if the assistant:

   A. centers the cuff directly over the artery.

   B. palpates the artery before beginning the procedure.

   C. inflates the cuff 80 mm Hg over the pulse level.

   D. chooses a cuff about 40% of the arm circumference.

3. Which of the following should be included in a nursing care plan for a patient with peripheral vascular disease?

   A. Dry the feet carefully by rubbing briskly.

   B. Buy shoes in the morning before swelling begins.

   C. Check the temperature of the water before stepping into the tub.

   D. Do not use powder on the feet.

4. You are caring for a patient who has had aortic surgery. You know to assess for signs of graft leakage. If all of the following are true, which would be considered the highest priority for nursing intervention?

   A. Hematoma at the incision

   B. Decreasing peripheral pulses

   C. Increased abdominal girth

   D. Decreasing blood pressure

5. The nurse is preparing a care plan for a patient with DVT. All of the following nursing diagnoses are appropriate EXCEPT:

   A. Pain, Acute.

   B. Ineffective Peripheral Tissue Perfusion.

   C. Impaired Skin Integrity.

   D. Risk for Constipation.

6. A patient, diagnosed with HTN, has been started on an ACE inhibitor. You know that the action of this medication to reduce blood pressure is by:

A. blocking the sympathetic input to the heart.

B. inhibiting the renin–angiotensin–aldosterone mechanism.

C. slowing the heart rate by reducing vasoconstriction.

D. relaxing vascular smooth muscle.

7. Your patient has a blood pressure of 164/100. You anticipate that the physician will:

A. recheck the BP in 1 year.

B. confirm the BP within 2 months.

C. refer for evaluation within 1 month.

D. refer for evaluation within 1 week.

8. You are teaching a patient about a diet low in vitamin K. You know that the patient understands the instructions because she tells you that:

A. "I will buy boxed macaroni and cheese instead of making it from scratch."

B. "I will eat lots of yogurt because I need the calcium."

C. "I will buy 1% milk from now on."

D. "I will stop buying spinach for a few months."

9. A 46-year-old executive asks you to help him understand how to reduce the stress in his life. He has recently been diagnosed with primary hypertension. Your best response should be:

A. "Stop worrying about everything."

B. "Exercise regularly every day."

C. "Take a class that focuses on therapeutic touch."

D. "Join a meditation group."

10. The primary manifestation of peripheral arterial disease is:

A. pain.

B. dependent rubor.

C. intermittent claudication.

D. decreased pulses.

11. A patient with DVT suddenly develops chest pain and SOB. The nurse suspects that this patient has developed:

A. an embolism.

B. atelectasis.

C. spontaneous pneumothorax.

D. bacterial pneumonia.

12. During the physical assessment, the nurse discovers that there are no palpable pedal pulses in the patient's left foot. Her next action should be to:

A. reattempt to palpate the pulses.

B. ask the charge nurse to palpate the pulses.

C. obtain a Doppler.

D. document the absent pulses.

13. A patient has been diagnosed with severe peripheral vascular disease. The nurse anticipates that the physician will order a low dose of aspirin. The rationale for the use of this medication is that aspirin:

   A. decreases the risk for clot formation.

   B. is an analgesic.

   C. can prevent a fever from occurring.

   D. is contraindicated in the patient with PVD.

14. You are discussing nursing interventions with the charge nurse for a patient with PVD. You suggest that the following intervention should be included:

   A. Gatch the knee at a 90-degree angle.

   B. Instruct the patient to keep the extremity in an independent position.

   C. Use a heating pad to keep the extremity warm.

   D. Assess the peripheral pulses every 4 hours.

15. The physician has prescribed the drug Coumadin for a patient with arterial disease. Which of the following should be included in the patient teaching?

   A. Increase the amount of vitamin K in the diet.

   B. Report any unusual bruises.

   C. Have blood levels of the medication taken every 6 months.

   D. Double the dose of the medication if a dose is skipped.

# CHAPTER 19

# The Hematologic and Lymphatic Systems and Assessment

## KEY TERMS

Match each term with its appropriate definition.

1. Plasma
2. Neutrophils
3. Erythrocytes
4. Hemoglobin
5. Purpura
6. Hemolysis
7. Lymphatic system
8. Leukocytes
9. Hemostasis
10. Platelets

A. An essential part of the body's clotting mechanism

B. Oxygen-carrying protein

C. A clear yellow, protein-rich fluid

D. Make up 50% to 70% of the circulating WBCs

E. Part of the body's defense against infection and disease

F. Includes lymphatic vessels, lymph nodes, and lymphoid organs

G. Shaped like biconcave disks

H. Purple rashes; caused by blood leaking into the skin

I. Blood clotting

J. The process of RBC destruction

## LEARNING OUTCOMES

1. What cells are suspended in plasma?
2. Describe *hemoglobin*.
3. Identify differential components in WBCs.
4. List three facts about platelets.
5. Describe the lymphatic system.
6. Identify lab tests used in lymphatic disorders.
7. Describe a bone marrow aspiration.
8. Identify the five stages in hemostasis.
9. Discuss the function of blood.
10. Identify the normal hemoglobin count in men and women.

# APPLY WHAT YOU LEARNED

A 38-year-old woman presents to the physician's office with complaints of fatigue, easy bruising, and a bruise on her leg that she states has been there for at least a month. Upon further assessment, she tells you that she sleeps as much as possible and cannot tolerate much activity. Her appetite is poor, and she is currently not taking any medications.

1. What diagnostic testing would the nurse expect with this patient?

2. What teaching would the nurse provide to the patient regarding some of the diagnostic testing?

# MULTIPLE CHOICE

Circle the answer that best completes the following statements.

1. A laboratory test used to diagnose hemolytic anemias and investigate transfusion reactions is called:
   A. electrophoresis.
   B. coagulation.
   C. Coombs'.
   D. Schilling.

2. Before a bone marrow aspiration, the nurse should have the patient:
   A. maintain a full bladder.
   B. lie in reverse Trendelenburg position.
   C. sign an informed consent.
   D. cough.

3. A patient is undergoing a biopsy to rule out malignancy of her left supraclavicular lymph node. The nurse tells her prior to the procedure:
   A. "You can't eat for 24 hours after the procedure."
   B. "You will bleed excessively following the procedure."
   C. "You are allowed only two visitors every 30 minutes."
   D. "I will monitor your vital signs routinely after the procedure."

4. The primary function of RBCs is to:
   A. transport oxygen to the cells.
   B. provide immunity to the body.
   C. destroy foreign matter.
   D. control bleeding.

5. Mr. Kelp is diagnosed with iron deficiency anemia. You should recommend a diet of increased:
   A. organ meats.
   B. fruits.
   C. bread.
   D. dairy products.

6. The nurse understands that the physician ordered an INR for a patient to:
   A. get more specific information about infections.
   B. to diagnose hemolytic anemias.
   C. evaluate warfarin therapy.
   D. measure the amount of iron stored in body tissues.

7. Mary, age 11, was diagnosed with leukemia. The nurse knows to watch for what observation in her assessment?
   A. Scales and rashes
   B. Petechiae and purpura
   C. Bowel and bladder control
   D. Loss of sensation

8. The most serious hazard for a patient who has had a bone marrow aspiration is:
   A. hemorrhage.
   B. pain.
   C. bruising.
   D. shock.

9. This evaluates the extrinsic clotting pathway, which is prolonged in Coumadin therapy:
   A. INR
   B. PTT
   C. PT
   D. APTT

10. A 28-year-old patient's transferrin lab value has come back slightly elevated. You ask her if she is taking:
    A. cocaine.
    B. amphetamines.
    C. Coumadin.
    D. oral contraceptives.

11. Normal ferritin for a woman should be in the range of:
    A. 10 to 310 ng/mL.
    B. 60 to 70 ng/mL.
    C. 15 to 445 ng/mL.
    D. 95 to 98 ng/mL.

12. RBCs have a life span of about:
    A. 30 days.
    B. 120 days.
    C. 45 days.
    D. 90 days.

13. WBCs are also called:
    A. platelets.
    B. erythrocytes.
    C. leukocytes.
    D. phagocytes.

14. The most plentiful of the WBCs are:
    A. granulocytes.
    B. eosinophils.
    C. basophils.
    D. monocytes.

15. What term is used to describe blood clotting?
    A. Hemostasis
    B. Hemocytoblastosis
    C. Erythrocytosis
    D. Homeostasis

# CHAPTER 20 ▶ Caring for Patients With Hematologic and Lymphatic Disorders

## KEY TERMS

Match each term with its appropriate definition.

1. Anemia
2. Polycythemia
3. Multiple myeloma
4. Leukemia
5. Purpura
6. Hemophilia
7. Stem cell transplant
8. Neutropenia
9. Malignant lymphomas
10. Thrombocytopenia

A. Hemorrhage into tissue

B. A group of malignant disorders of WBCs

C. Hemoglobin concentration, or the number of circulating RBCs, is decreased

D. A group of hereditary clotting factor deficiencies

E. A platelet count of less than 100,000 platelets per milliliter of blood

F. Condition characterized by lymphocyte proliferation

G. May be used along with chemotherapy or radiation to treat some types of leukemia

H. Excess erythropoietin production

I. Malignancy in which plasma cells multiply uncontrollably and infiltrate bone marrow, lymph nodes, and other tissues

J. Decrease in the number of circulating neutrophils

## LEARNING OUTCOMES

1. List several manifestations of anemia.
2. Describe *thalassemia*.
3. Identify dietary sources of folic acid.
4. What is the focus of treatment for polycythemia?
5. Describe manifestations of leukemia.
6. Identify the four major classifications of leukemia.
7. Identify nursing diagnoses involved with leukemia.
8. Define *agranulocytosis*.
9. Describe *thrombocytopenia*.
10. Identify risk factors for disseminated intravascular coagulation.

## APPLY WHAT YOU LEARNED

Upon assessment of a new patient on your wing, you discover enlarged lymph nodes and a fever. When talking to the patient, you find out that he has been having night sweats, fatigue, and weight loss. He also complains about itchy skin and malaise. The patient tells you that this has been going on for a few weeks.

1. What would these manifestations mean in terms of diagnosis?
2. What treatment options are available for this patient?
3. What nursing diagnoses apply to this situation?

## MULTIPLE CHOICE

Circle the answer that best completes the following statements.

1. Acquired hemolytic anemia results when RBCs are damaged by outside factors, such as:
   A. immune responses.
   B. cellular development.
   C. healing.
   D. stress.

2. Aplastic anemia may follow injury to stem cells in bone marrow caused by:
   A. certain infections.
   B. drugs or radiation.
   C. chemicals.
   D. all of the above.

3. Aplastic anemia, if left untreated, could ultimately lead to:
   A. leukocytosis.
   B. leukopenia.
   C. nothing; it corrects itself.
   D. heart failure.

4. Sickle cell anemia usually affects people of:
   A. Mediterranean descent.
   B. Asian descent.
   C. African descent.
   D. European descent.

5. Myelodysplastic syndrome (MDS) is a group of stem cell disorders characterized by abnormal-appearing bone marrow and ineffective blood cell production. It is primarily a disorder of:
   A. middle adults.
   B. young adults.
   C. older adults.
   D. children.

6. After an autologous bone marrow transplant, the risk of death is greater for a patient due to:
    A. microorganisms.
    B. bleeding.
    C. immunosuppression.
    D. pain.

7. An alternative to bone marrow transplant is:
    A. brain cell transplant.
    B. stem cell transplant.
    C. spinal fluid transplant.
    D. all of the above.

8. The inheritance patterns for both hemophilia A and B are:
    A. Y-linked recessive disorders.
    B. X-linked recessive disorders.
    C. female reproductive disorders.
    D. male reproductive disorders.

9. A person with Hodgkin lymphoma may have a nursing diagnosis of:
    A. Risk for Impaired Skin Integrity.
    B. Disturbed Thought Processes.
    C. Deficient Fluid Volume.
    D. none of the above.

10. Exposure to environmental toxins such as radiation and benzene and cancer treatment with radiation and chemotherapy are identified risk factors for:
    A. AIDS.
    B. BMT.
    C. SCT.
    D. MDS.

11. A condition where the concentration of hemoglobin is decreased is known as:
    A. anemia.
    B. amenorrhea.
    C. anorexia.
    D. agranulocytosis.

12. People receiving PN may develop a deficiency in:
    A. glucose.
    B. chloride.
    C. folate.
    D. lipids.

13. Thalassemia usually affects which group?
   A. Hispanics
   B. Caucasians
   C. Mediterranean
   D. Canadians

14. Dietary sources of iron include all of the following EXCEPT:
   A. beef.
   B. pork.
   C. cheese.
   D. potatoes.

15. An excessively high red blood cell count is known as:
   A. polycythemia.
   B. leukemia.
   C. anemia.
   D. thalassemia.

# CHAPTER 21 ▶ The Respiratory System and Assessment

## KEY TERMS

Match each term with its appropriate definition.

1. Compliance
2. Respiration
3. Nares
4. Nasopharynx
5. Epiglottis
6. Larynx
7. Barrel chest
8. Sinuses
9. Ventilation
10. Adventitious

A. Located between laryngopharynx and trachea

B. Increased anterior–posterior chest diameter

C. Abnormal breath sounds

D. Contains the tonsils and adenoids

E. Process that provides oxygen to the cells of the body and eliminates carbon dioxide

F. Openings in facial bones that lighten the skull

G. Breathing; air moves into and out of the lungs

H. External opening of the nasal cavity

I. Distensibility of the lungs; depends on both lung tissue and rib cage

J. Closes during swallowing to prevent aspiration

## LEARNING OUTCOMES

1. Describe the function of the upper respiratory system.
2. Identify the structures of the upper respiratory system.
3. Describe the function of the lower respiratory system.
4. Identify the structures of the lower respiratory system.
5. Discuss the respiratory changes associated with aging.
6. Define *adventitious breath sounds*.
7. Describe *pulse oximetry*.
8. Describe the procedure to obtain a throat swab.
9. Identify the purpose of the ventilation-perfusion scan.
10. Discuss patient and family teaching regarding bronchoscopy procedures.

## APPLY WHAT YOU LEARNED

A 72-year-old male presents to the clinic with complaints of "flu-like symptoms." He tells you that he has had a sore throat for the past 4 days with a dry, nonproductive cough. The patient denies allergies and chronic illness.

1. Describe the nursing assessment that will be performed for this patient.
2. What diagnostic testing would the nurse expect to see ordered by the physician?
3. What other pertinent data would the nurse ask the patient in reference to the "flu-like symptoms"?

## MULTIPLE CHOICE

Circle the answer that best completes the following statements.

1. The primary laboratory tests used to evaluate the respiratory system and diagnose the disorders affecting it are:
   A. tissue biopsy, pulse oximetry, and arterial blood gases.
   B. arterial blood gases; tissue biopsy; and nasal, throat, and sputum cultures.
   C. nasal, throat, and sputum cultures; ear swab; tissue biopsy.
   D. tissue biopsy, arterial blood gases, and blood glucose.

2. The nurse knows that when obtaining a sputum culture, it is important to do what following the procedure?
   A. Use aseptic technique.
   B. Instruct the patient to cough several times.
   C. Provide mouth care.
   D. Perform tracheal suctioning.

3. Lung volume and capacity are measured with:
   A. LCDs.
   B. PETs.
   C. LATs.
   D. PFTs.

4. You are teaching a patient going for a pulmonary function test to stop using bronchodilators, drinking caffeinated beverages, or smoking 4–6 hours before the test because:
   A. the patient could die.
   B. the testing policy dictates.
   C. bronchodilators, smoking, and caffeine interfere with test results.
   D. the results will always be positive.

5. Marta, age 25, has asthma. She uses a peak expiratory flow rate (PEFR) meter on a day-to-day basis to:
   A. monitor air humidity.
   B. assess her breathing pattern.
   C. monitor airway constriction.
   D. balance the amount of rest periods and activities.

6. Jason, age 38, was diagnosed with laryngeal tumors via:
   A. laryngoscopy.
   B. bronchoscopy.
   C. EGD.
   D. EEG.

7. A patent airway and unobstructed airflow are vital to sustain life and:
   A. well-being.
   B. lung capacity.
   C. function.
   D. love.

8. Before doing a CT of the head and neck, an important nursing implication is to ask about:
   A. consent.
   B. next of kin.
   C. bleeding.
   D. allergies.

9. Following arterial puncture, the nurse often is responsible for applying pressure to the site for a period of:
   A. at least 5 minutes.
   B. 30 minutes.
   C. 2 to 5 minutes.
   D. 1 hour.

10. A detergent-like substance that helps keep alveoli open is called:
    A. mainstem.
    B. hilus.
    C. surfactant.
    D. bronchus.

11. During inspiration, the diaphragm:
    A. contracts and flattens out.
    B. dilates and fills out.
    C. constricts and releases gases.
    D. holds on to air.

12. In a patient with barrel chest, the chest is:
    A. decreased in anterior–posterior diameter.
    B. increased in anterior–posterior diameter.
    C. symmetrical in diameter.
    D. concave in diameter.

13. The pharynx is a passageway for:

   **A.** air and food.

   **B.** bile and mucus.

   **C.** singing and talking.

   **D.** bronchi.

14. The nasopharynx starts at the:

   **A.** mouth.

   **B.** tongue.

   **C.** nose.

   **D.** throat.

15. The double-layered membrane that covers the lungs is called:

   **A.** pleura.

   **B.** bronchi.

   **C.** rales.

   **D.** trachea.

# CHAPTER **22** ▶ *Caring for Patients With Upper Respiratory Disorders*

## KEY TERMS

Match each term with its appropriate definition.

1. Rhinitis
2. Influenza
3. Sinusitis
4. Pharyngitis
5. Tonsillitis
6. Sleep apnea
7. Stridor
8. Epistaxis
9. Dysphagia
10. Tracheostomy

A. Temporary absence of breathing during sleep

B. A highly contagious viral respiratory disease

C. Difficulty swallowing

D. Inflammation of the nasal cavities

E. Inflammation of the mucous membranes of the sinuses

F. Acute inflammation of the tonsils

G. A high-pitched, harsh sound heard during inspiration

H. Surgical opening in the trachea

I. Acute inflammation of the throat

J. Nosebleed

## LEARNING OUTCOMES

1. Identify the manifestations of acute pharyngitis.
2. Describe the course and possible complications of rhinitis and influenza.
3. Describe people who should receive annual influenza vaccines.
4. Describe the methods of nursing care in controlling URIs in long-term care.
5. List several complementary therapies and practices used to treat many URIs.
6. Identify some nursing diagnoses of patients with URIs.
7. Describe *pertussis*.
8. Identify the medications used with epistaxis.
9. Identify the manifestations of nasal fractures.
10. Describe *sleep apnea*.

## APPLY WHAT YOU LEARNED

A 61-year-old man presents to the clinic for follow-up regarding his diagnosis of laryngeal cancer. He continues to smoke 2 ppd and drinks three to four alcoholic beverages per day. His voice is hoarse, and he complaints of a sore throat and decreased appetite. Total laryngectomy is suggested at this time by the physician.

1. How would the nurse explain the importance of abstaining from alcohol (ETOH) and cigarettes?
2. Describe teaching regarding a total laryngectomy.
3. Discuss postoperative care for this patient.

## MULTIPLE CHOICE

Circle the answer that best completes the following statements.

1. Before administering the polyvalent influenza virus vaccine to a patient, the nurse should:
   A. ask the patient about previous flu episodes.
   B. obtain vital signs.
   C. note the patient's allergies to eggs.
   D. request the patient to sign an informed consent.

2. The patient who is receiving antibiotics for a bacterial infection is no longer contagious after:
   A. 12 hours.
   B. 24 hours.
   C. 48 hours.
   D. 72 hours.

3. Which of the following medications, if used longer than 3 to 5 days, may result in rebound congestion?
   A. Fexofenadine
   B. Neo-Synephrine
   C. Clesmastine
   D. Allegra

4. You are assigned to assist in writing the discharge plans for a patient who has had endoscopic sinus surgery. Patient teaching should include:
   A. sneeze into a tissue to prevent spreading of microorganisms.
   B. no lifting restrictions for 3 days.
   C. avoid smoking.
   D. notify the physician for a temperature greater than 100°F.

5. Nursing interventions for the diagnosis of Ineffective Airway Clearance should include:
   A. balance the amount of rest periods and activities.
   B. assess the patient's sleep patterns.
   C. monitor the cough reflex.
   D. instruct the patient in the use of throat lozenges.

6. Posterior nosebleeds are usually associated with secondary systemic disorders. The individual most affected by this form of epistaxis is the:

   A. 30-year-old football player.

   B. 62-year-old housewife.

   C. 14-year-old ballet dancer.

   D. 76-year-old retired engineer.

7. Appropriate first aid for the patient with an anterior nosebleed includes:

   A. pinching the nose away from the septum.

   B. applying ice packs to the nose.

   C. sitting position, leaning slightly backward.

   D. tilting the head upward.

8. The most commonly broken bone of the face is the:

   A. mandible.

   B. maxilla.

   C. nose.

   D. temporal bone.

9. Your patient has undergone rhinoplasty and will be discharged from the hospital in 2 days. He is anxious about the swelling and bruising on his face and asks how long the bruises will be noticeable. You reply that this condition should subside in:

   A. 3 to 5 days.

   B. 6 to 10 days.

   C. 10 to 14 days.

   D. several months.

10. The most common cause of airway obstruction in the adult is:

    A. swollen tongue.

    B. drowning.

    C. anaphylactic shock.

    D. food lodged in the throat.

11. The term used to describe a high-pitched, wheezing sound created by an airway obstruction is:

    A. crowing.

    B. stridor.

    C. sonorous.

    D. crepitus.

12. Laryngeal tumors can be:

    A. in the glottis, the supraglottis, or the subglottis.

    B. benign or malignant.

    C. slow growing.

    D. all of the above.

13. Laryngeal cancer may be caused by several factors. The risk factor that is considered to be the most modifiable is:

    **A.** gender.

    **B.** age.

    **C.** nutrition.

    **D.** use of alcohol and tobacco.

14. The nurse knows her teaching about tracheostomy care to the nursing student has been effective when the student says:

    **A.** "I will work quickly, making sure to keep my gloves clean so that I don't have to stop and change them during the procedure."

    **B.** "I know it is important to use sterile technique when suctioning."

    **C.** "I will assess the patient's lung sounds only after I suction."

    **D.** "I will clean the incision with soap and water."

15. What is the most important measure to reduce the risk of influenza?

    **A.** Yearly immunization

    **B.** Vitamin C every day

    **C.** Proper hand hygiene

    **D.** Antiviral drugs

# CHAPTER 23

# *Caring for Patients With Lower Respiratory Disorders*

## KEY TERMS

Match each term with its appropriate definition.

1. Atelectasis
2. Dyspnea
3. Hemothorax
4. Acute respiratory distress syndrome
5. Cyanosis
6. Chronic obstructive pulmonary disease
7. Asthma
8. Pneumothorax
9. Pulmonary hypertension
10. Hemoptysis

A. Blood in the pleural space; usually results from chest trauma or surgery

B. Bluish-gray skin color

C. Partial or total lung collapse and airlessness; may be acute or chronic

D. Accumulation of air in the pleural space

E. Difficulty breathing

F. Inflammatory respiratory disease characterized by chronic and progressive obstruction of airflow in the lungs

G. Bloody sputum

H. Chronic inflammatory disorder of the airways characterized by recurrent episodes of wheezing, breathlessness, chest tightness, and coughing

I. Abnormal elevation of the pulmonary arterial pressure

J. Severe form of acute respiratory failure; characterized by inflammatory pulmonary edema and unresponsive progressive hypoxemia

## LEARNING OUTCOMES

1. Define *bronchitis*, *emphysema*, and *pneumonia*.
2. Describe *aspiration pneumonia*.
3. Identify diagnostic testing for pneumonia.
4. Identify nursing diagnoses for pneumonia.
5. Describe *tuberculosis*.
6. Define negative and positive TB test results.
7. Identify several measures that can be taken to prevent asthma.
8. Describe manifestations of COPD.
9. Define *barrel chest*.
10. Identify manifestations of lung cancer.

## APPLY WHAT YOU LEARNED

A 59-year-old woman on your unit has been diagnosed with a pneumothorax and will have a chest tube inserted for treatment. The patient has chronic lung disease and has recently quit smoking. She has family members present who are very supportive and eager to learn how to help.

1. Describe nursing care regarding the chest tube.
2. What nursing diagnoses would the nurse apply to this patient?
3. What types of evaluation would the nurse provide?

## MULTIPLE CHOICE

Circle the answer that best completes the following statements.

1. The most common cause of chronic obstructive pulmonary disease is:
   A. environmental pollutants.
   B. alpha-1 antitrypsin deficiency.
   C. heredity.
   D. smoking.

2. A nursing assistant asks you why the lower respiratory system is so important. She understands that you have to breathe in order to live but wants to know the physiology. Your best response would be:
   A. "The lower respiratory tract warms the air."
   B. "The bronchi allow carbon dioxide and oxygen exchange."
   C. "The alveoli produce a substance that helps the lungs move freely."
   D. "Oxygen and carbon dioxide exchange helps to regulate the acid–base balance."

3. The nurse is teaching the patient about her asthmatic condition. The focus of the nursing plan should be:
   A. preventing death.
   B. controlling symptoms.
   C. preventing the asthma attack.
   D. instructing about the pathophysiology of asthma as a disease.

4. The patient with asthma is being evaluated for Ineffective Airway Clearance. Which of the following nursing interventions should be the nurse's highest priority?
   A. Monitor oxygen saturation level.
   B. Check the chart for the latest ABG report.
   C. Assess respiratory effort.
   D. Check the amount and color of sputum.

5. Your patient is complaining of SOB. As you begin your assessment, you note that only the right side of the chest is moving. Your next action should be to:
   A. call the charge nurse.
   B. ask the patient why she is breathing on only one side.
   C. apply oxygen at 3 L/nc.
   D. auscultate both lungs.

6. A patient was working in a factory that produces a variety of glues. He presents to the emergency room with SOB, fever, and chest pain. Based on your knowledge of pneumonia, you anticipate that this patient might have:

    A. aspiration pneumonia.

    B. *Pneumocystis jiroveci* pneumonia.

    C. tuberculosis.

    D. noninfectious pneumonia.

7. Mr. Jackson will be having a thoracentesis on your shift. If all of the following are appropriate interventions for the patient before the procedure, which would have the highest priority?

    A. Tell the patient that some pressure will be felt.

    B. Bring the supplies to the bedside.

    C. Administer a cough suppressant, if ordered.

    D. Reinforce teaching about the procedure.

8. The nurse is reading the TB skin test for a patient. She measures the redness as 6 mm. This measurement is:

    A. a negative response.

    B. a negative response with no infection.

    C. positive for a person with HIV.

    D. invalid because the induration was not read.

9. Johnny, a 29-year-old patient with HIV, has been taking INH for 2 months. He is now complaining of numbness in his feet. You explain that:

    A. this is an unusual side effect.

    B. you will note this in his record and let the physician know right away.

    C. it is a minor problem and will resolve over time.

    D. it is probably caused by his HIV status.

10. A second-day postoperative patient complains of sudden chest pain and SOB. The nurse suspects:

    A. pulmonary embolism.

    B. aspiration pneumonia.

    C. atelectasis.

    D. hemorrhage.

11. You are assessing the chest tube for a patient with lung cancer. You notice that the water in the water seal is fluctuating with the patient's breathing. Your next action should be to:

    A. continue with the assessment.

    B. call the physician after your assessment.

    C. ask the patient if he feels okay.

    D. shake the water chamber to stop the bubbling.

12. A 16-year-old male is brought to the emergency room with a severe headache, nausea, and SOB. His skin has a cherry red appearance. You immediately realize that this patient may be experiencing:

    A. carbon monoxide poisoning.

    B. status asthmaticus.

    C. walking pneumonia.

    D. cystic fibrosis.

13. During a football game, a player trips and falls. He is brought to the local clinic complaining of severe SOB, tachypnea, and pallor. You note there is asymmetrical lung expansion. You anticipate the insertion of a(n):

   A. IV line.

   B. Foley catheter.

   C. chest tube.

   D. endotracheal tube.

14. The physician has ordered a sputum sample. The nurse knows that the best time to obtain a sputum sample is:

   A. after the first dose of the antibiotic.

   B. right before bedtime.

   C. early in the morning.

   D. late in the afternoon.

15. You are preparing to suction a tracheostomy patient. You remember from your respiratory class that you can apply suction for:

   A. 10 seconds.

   B. 15 seconds.

   C. 25 seconds.

   D. 30 seconds.

# 24 ▶ The Gastrointestinal System and Assessment

## KEY TERMS

Match each term with its appropriate definition.

| | |
|---|---|
| 1. Hepatocytes | A. Basic functional units of the liver |
| 2. Peristalsis | B. Partially digested food mixed with gastric juices |
| 3. Metabolism | C. Organic, essential nutrients |
| 4. Chyme | D. Alternating waves of contraction and relaxation; allows the esophagus to carry food to the stomach |
| 5. Vitamins | E. Liver cells |
| 6. Lobules | F. Substances in foods that are used by the body for growth, maintenance, and repair |
| 7. Nutrition | |
| 8. Nutrients | G. Biochemical reactions that occur in the cells; involves anabolism and catabolism |
| 9. Carbohydrates | H. Area behind the stomach and the peritoneal membrane |
| 10. Retroperitoneal | I. Composed of simple or complex sugars |
| | J. Process of ingesting, absorbing, using, and eliminating food in the body |

## LEARNING OUTCOMES

1. List four specialized types of cells in the stomach lining.
2. Explain the components of the gastrointestinal tract.
3. Describe the functions of the liver.
4. Identify the purpose of an upper endoscopy.
5. Discuss the rationale for using imaging studies for gastrointestinal complaints.
6. Describe the diagnostic test called esophageal manometry.
7. List the organs located in the right upper quadrant of the abdomen.
8. Identify the purpose of the stool specimen test for ova and parasites.
9. Describe manifestations related to vitamin and mineral deficiencies.
10. Identify symptoms associated with water deficits and excesses.

## APPLY WHAT YOU LEARNED

A 45-year-old male presents to your unit with complaints of abdominal pain that has been progressing over the last 4 days. He states that he has had diarrhea for about a week and does not really have an appetite.

1. What types of questions should the nurse ask to assess the situation further?
2. In what order would the nurse assess the abdomen?
3. What diagnostic testing would the nurse expect the physician to order?
4. Would the nurse offer this patient anything to eat?

## MULTIPLE CHOICE

Circle the answer that best completes the following statements.

1. A patient suffering from multiple dental caries states, "I've been dieting a lot lately." What type of diet is this patient likely on?
   A. High carbohydrates
   B. Low fat
   C. High protein
   D. Fasting

2. Dianne, a patient in the hospital, has not eaten well in several days. She and her boyfriend broke up before she entered the hospital. The nurse realizes that emotions such as stress or anxiety affect the GI tract by:
   A. increasing gastric secretions.
   B. neutralizing stomach acid.
   C. inhibiting gastric motility.
   D. excreting bile.

3. The nurse understands that which of the following is NOT a gastrointestinal change associated with aging?
   A. Increased gastric emptying time
   B. Constipation
   C. Increased acid production
   D. Fewer taste buds

4. A gastric analysis includes which of the following?
   A. Allowing the patient to smoke
   B. Inserting an NG tube
   C. Observing for falls
   D. Comparing preanalysis weight

5. The nurse understands that the small intestine is where:
   A. chyme is produced.
   B. indigestible food residue is eliminated from the body.
   C. bile is produced.
   D. food is chemically digested and absorbed.

6. Corey was admitted with diarrhea and dehydration. He had at least four foul-smelling, mucous-filled loose stools every 3 hours. You know the physician will order a(n):

    A. serum albumin level.

    B. gastric lavage.

    C. endoscopy.

    D. specimen for ova and parasites.

7. The nurse is explaining to a patient why the physician has ordered a stool for occult blood. The best explanation would be:

    A. "It is used to assess general nutritional status and liver function."

    B. "It is used to assess for gastrointestinal bleeding."

    C. "Don't worry about it right now. You're probably fine."

    D. "It is used to detect the presence of infective organisms."

8. Mr. Lee, an 89-year-old patient who rarely eats his meals, is losing weight. The nurse knows to assess:

    A. mucous membranes and gums.

    B. food tolerance.

    C. A and B.

    D. the soft palate.

9. Ms. Ray has soft, spoon-shaped nails. The nurse is aware that this is due to:

    A. protein deficiency.

    B. high-fat diet.

    C. smoking.

    D. iron deficiency.

10. Mrs. Matherly is returning to your unit following a lower GI series. Which of the following nursing interventions is the most important?

    A. Encourage fluids.

    B. Monitor for pain.

    C. Provide detailed postop instructions.

    D. Encourage splinting.

11. Which of the following vitamins is water soluble?

    A. A

    B. D

    C. E

    D. B

12. Energy that is produced by food is measured in:

    A. metabolic rates.

    B. kilocalories.

    C. resting metabolic rates.

    D. body surface area.

13. When assessing the abdomen, which task is performed first?

   A. Percussion

   B. Palpation

   C. Auscultation

   D. Injection

14. AST and ALT are used to evaluate:

   A. gastric function.

   B. pancreas function.

   C. liver function.

   D. respiratory function.

15. Which diagnostic test is used to detect bleeding in the peritoneal cavity?

   A. Esophageal manometry

   B. Paracentesis

   C. Barium enema

   D. CT scans

# 25 ▶ Caring for Patients With Nutritional and Upper Gastrointestinal Disorders

## KEY TERMS

Match each term with its appropriate definition.

1. Anorexia
2. Hematemesis
3. Anastomosis
4. Obesity
5. Malnutrition
6. Melena
7. Nausea
8. Borborygmi
9. Dysphagia
10. Peptic ulcer

A. Excess adipose tissue or fat

B. Loud, hyperactive bowel sounds

C. Bloody emesis

D. Pain or difficulty swallowing

E. Surgical connection

F. Loss of appetite

G. Poor nourishment from improper diet or metabolic defect

H. Blood in the stool

I. Break in the mucous lining of the stomach or duodenum where it comes in contact with gastric juice

J. Vague but unpleasant sensation of sickness or queasiness

## LEARNING OUTCOMES

1. Define upper-body and lower-body obesity.
2. Identify some problems associated with obesity.
3. Describe behavior strategies for weight loss.
4. Discuss conditions associated with malnutrition.
5. Define *catabolism*.
6. Explain the purpose of enteral feedings.
7. Describe *anorexia nervosa*.
8. Define *stomatitis*.
9. Identify manifestations of oral cancer.
10. Describe *gastroesophageal reflux*.

## APPLY WHAT YOU LEARNED

A patient comes to you stating that she is prepared to have a gastric bypass to assist with weight loss and to improve her overall health. The patient is categorized as morbidly obese and qualifies for the procedure. The patient has documentation from a dietician regarding past weight loss efforts. The patient has also been screened by a psychiatrist to rule out disordered eating and thinking.

1. What educational topics must the nurse discuss with the patient before the surgeon obtains consent?
2. What side effects should the nurse explain to the patient regarding aftercare?
3. What would be the priorities in nursing care regarding this patient?

## MULTIPLE CHOICE

Circle the answer that best completes the following statements.

1. A patient suffering from bulimia is at risk for:
   A. weight gain.
   B. diarrhea.
   C. esophageal damage.
   D. hyperglycemia.

2. Johnny is going to be receiving enteral tube feedings for a period of time. You know that enteral feedings may be administered through:
   A. nasogastric and gastric tubes.
   B. gastric and cecum tubes.
   C. gastric tubes only.
   D. nasogastric, gastrostomy, and jejunostomy tubes.

3. The nurse is caring for a stroke patient receiving enteral feeding via NG tube of 120 mL Ensure/hr. Her main concern at this time would be prevention of:
   A. diarrhea.
   B. aspiration.
   C. nasal irritation.
   D. constipation.

4. A patient receiving PN would be expected to have daily blood specimens drawn for:
   A. calcium.
   B. glucose.
   C. sodium.
   D. potassium.

5. The nurse knows her teaching has been understood when the patient says:

A. "My BMI is 23, so I know I am at a healthy weight."

B. "Now that I know my BMI is 23, I will go on a diet and exercise every day so that I can lose weight."

C. "My BMI of 23 lets me know that my central obesity is ok."

D. "My BMI is 23, so I know I am at higher risk for hypertension."

6. Maxine was admitted with acute gastritis. During her morning bath, she suddenly begins to throw up blood. Your first action should be to:

A. administer prescribed antiemetic.

B. raise the head of the bed.

C. increase the IV fluid rate.

D. call the physician.

7. You are explaining to a patient who has been diagnosed with peptic ulcer disease the effects that cigarette smoking has on the stomach. Your best explanation might be:

A. "The tar in the cigarette coats the lining of the stomach."

B. "Smoking increases the production of gastric acid secretion."

C. "Cigarettes inhibit bicarbonate secretion."

D. "The nicotine increases blood flow to the gastric mucosa."

8. Mr. Jessup tells you that he becomes nauseated about 10 minutes after he has eaten. In addition, he states that his stomach cramps and makes loud noises. To alleviate some of these symptoms, the nurse would suggest which of the following?

A. Eat two large meals a day.

B. Drink lots of water with the food.

C. Rest in a recumbent position after eating.

D. Increase the amount of simple sugars in the diet.

9. The nurse is aware that there is an increased risk for stomach cancer in patients who:

A. eat diets high in fiber.

B. have been diagnosed with *H. pylori* gastritis.

C. are under a lot of stress.

D. smoke two packs of cigarettes per day.

10. Mrs. Elliot is returning to your unit following an endoscopy. Which of the following nursing interventions is the most important?

A. Withhold fluids until the gag reflex returns.

B. Monitor for pain.

C. Provide detailed discharge instructions.

D. Discourage coughing.

11. You are performing a gastric lavage and have suctioned 135 mL of fluid from the stomach. Your initial irrigation was 100 mL of water. On the I&O record you will document:

    A. 135 mL gastric contents.

    B. 235 mL gastric contents and lavage.

    C. 35 mL gastric contents.

    D. 100 mL gastric contents.

12. Mrs. Tubbman has a new gastrostomy tube that is going to be used for the first time. You are unable to aspirate any stomach contents. Bowel sounds are absent. Your next action is to:

    A. use the tube because the x-ray verified placement.

    B. hold the tube feeding until the doctor makes rounds.

    C. call the doctor and inform her of your findings.

    D. ask the charge nurse to begin the feedings.

13. You are teaching a patient about the use of metoclopramide. Which of the following is NOT true concerning this medication?

    A. It may cause drowsiness.

    B. It is used to prevent dizzy spells.

    C. Adverse reactions with alcohol have been documented.

    D. It may have a side effect of muscle tremors.

14. The school nurse is seeing an 18-year-old girl for complaints of fatigue. The patient states that her vitamins "just don't seem to work." She appears unusually thin. The nurse believes that the patient needs further teaching because:

    A. teenagers are not nutritionally educated.

    B. teen girls are at risk for poor nutrition due to societal expectations.

    C. she is on the basketball team and weight loss is expected.

    D. she is not taking the proper amount of vitamins.

15. Measures that are used to evaluate obesity include:

    A. BMI.

    B. insulin resistance.

    C. serum electrolyte levels.

    D. all of the above.

# CHAPTER 26 ▸ Caring for Patients With Bowel Disorders

## KEY TERMS

Match each term with its appropriate definition.

1. Diverticulitis
2. Ileostomy
3. Colostomy
4. Diarrhea
5. Colectomy
6. Crohn disease
7. Ulcerative colitis
8. Laparoscopy
9. Laparotomy
10. Paralytic ileus

A. Ostomy in the ileum of the small intestine

B. Chronic, relapsing inflammatory disorder that can affect any part of the GI tract from the mouth to the anus

C. Ostomy made in the colon

D. Chronic inflammatory disorder involving the mucosal layers of the colon and rectum

E. Inflammation and perforation of a diverticulum, usually in the sigmoid colon

F. Increase in the frequency, volume, and water content of stool

G. Exploration of the abdomen using an endoscope

H. Occurs when peristalsis slows or stops

I. Surgical removal of the colon

J. Surgical opening of the abdomen

## LEARNING OUTCOMES

1. Describe the pathophysiology of diarrhea.
2. Identify foods that may aggravate chronic diarrhea.
3. Discuss preventive measures for constipation in the older adult.
4. Describe the various types of enemas.
5. Define *IBS*.
6. Discuss nursing care regarding a small bowel series.
7. Define *malabsorption*.
8. Describe the manifestations of peritonitis.
9. Discuss the diagnostic testing for Crohn disease.
10. Identify risk factors for colorectal cancer.

## APPLY WHAT YOU LEARNED

A patient is seen for a follow-up due to a recent hospitalization for IBD. She states that she is feeling better and is slowly advancing her diet from liquids to soft foods that are low in fat. She currently denies diarrhea, constipation, and pain. Upon assessment, you notice that her abdomen is slightly distended and her blood pressure is 110/78.

1. What nursing diagnoses would apply to this patient?
2. Based on the given information, is this normal or abnormal? Why or why not?
3. Explain some teaching the nurse could provide to this patient.

## MULTIPLE CHOICE

Circle the answer that best completes the following statements.

1. The nurse is changing an ostomy pouch. Which of the following should be completed first?
   A. Note the color of the stoma and surrounding skin.
   B. Use a measuring guide to check the stoma size.
   C. Remove the soiled pouch.
   D. Cleanse the skin with soap and water.

2. You are assisting an older patient in filling out the diet menu. The patient has chronic diarrhea. Which of the following items should NOT be ordered for this patient?
   A. Apple juice
   B. Roast beef
   C. Green beans
   D. Spaghetti

3. The nurse understands that the patient needs reinforcement of her teaching about his low-residue diet for a colostomy when he says:
   A. "I'll juice my vegetables rather than eating them raw."
   B. "I will eat brown rice and barley."
   C. "I will replace my usual apple with some juice."
   D. "When I make my famous potato salad next week, I'll be sure to leave the peels on the potatoes."

4. A young patient asks the nurse what can cause constipation. The best response is:
   A. lack of exercise.
   B. chronic laxative use.
   C. voluntary suppression of the urge.
   D. all of the above.

5. A patient is preparing for a colonoscopy. The physician orders magnesium citrate. Which of the following statements, if made by the patient, would indicate an understanding of your teaching instructions?
   A. "I'll take the medication at bedtime so it has time to work."
   B. "I keep the drink at room temperature so it will taste better."
   C. "This medication will give me some cramps."
   D. "It's okay to eat breakfast at 6 A.M., since my exam isn't until 8 A.M."

6. An older patient has been taking mineral oil as a laxative routinely for several months. The nurse can expect that this patient will have a deficiency of:

   A. vitamin A.

   B. vitamin C.

   C. vitamin B.

   D. vitamin F.

7. When preparing a patient for a sigmoidoscopy, the teaching plan should include which of the following instructions?

   A. Sterile water may be injected into the bowel for better visualization.

   B. The patient will be placed in the prone position.

   C. No food or water can be consumed 8 hours before the test.

   D. A clear liquid diet is ordered for 2 to 3 days before the examination.

8. What is the priority area of focus for the nursing care of patients undergoing nonsurgical treatment for bowel obstruction?

   A. Providing pain relief

   B. Teaching about a healthy diet

   C. Assessing for anxiety

   D. Preventing complications of obstruction and surgery

9. Which of the following patients is at high risk for developing colon cancer?

   A. A 58-year-old male diagnosed with prostate cancer

   B. A 24-year-old female with a family history of ovarian cancer

   C. A 37-year-old male with inflammatory bowel disease

   D. A 16-year-old female with morbid obesity

10. A patient tells you that his colostomy bag odor is embarrassing and asks you what he can do to minimize this problem. Your best response would be:

    A. "Be sure to eat lots of cabbage and eggs."

    B. "There's not much that we can do about the smell."

    C. "There are odor tablets that you can put in the bag."

    D. "I don't think the smell is so bad. Don't worry about it."

11. Which observation of a patient who has a nursing diagnosis of Risk for Impaired Skin Integrity would indicate that the outcome is successful?

    A. The patient has developed a small, 2-cm reddened area on his sacrum.

    B. The patient has a small rash on the perineal area.

    C. The patient's skin is intact.

    D. The patient requires aloe vera cream for the lesion on buttocks.

12. When a patient has a nursing diagnosis of Risk for Deficient Fluid Volume, which of the following nursing interventions should be included in the care plan?

    A. Maintain accurate intake and output records.

    B. Record the patient's weight weekly.

    C. Assess for signs of dehydration, such as moist skin.

    D. Document the vital signs every shift.

13. Which of the following nursing diagnoses would be the most appropriate for a patient with colon cancer?

   A. Acute Pain

   B. Grieving

   C. Risk for Sexual Dysfunction

   D. Risk for Impaired Skin Integrity

14. A patient is being discharged from the hospital with a new ostomy appliance. Prior to discharge, it is important to request a referral to the:

   A. dietician.

   B. home health nurse.

   C. ostomy and wound care nurse.

   D. physical therapist.

15. A 24-year-old patient is admitted to the surgical floor with excruciating pain in the right groin. He is nauseated and has vomited 300 mL of yellow bile. Visible inspection reveals a mass in the groin. The medical diagnosis for this patient might be:

   A. ventral hernia.

   B. strangulated hernia.

   C. umbilical hernia.

   D. incisional hernia.

# CHAPTER 27

# Caring for Patients With Gallbladder, Liver, and Pancreatic Disorders

## KEY TERMS

Match each term with its appropriate definition.

1. Esophageal varices
2. Cirrhosis
3. Paracentesis
4. Hepatitis
5. Hepatic encephalopathy
6. Ascites
7. Portal hypertension
8. Hepatorenal syndrome
9. Jaundice
10. Icteric

A. Can be caused when blood is shunted around the congested liver, allowing toxic waste products to accumulate

B. Collateral vessels that develop in the distal esophagus

C. Inflammation of the liver

D. Type of acute kidney failure that occurs when blood flow to the kidneys is affected by portal hypertension

E. Yellow staining of tissues that occurs when bilirubin is not metabolized and excreted

F. Chronic liver disease that destroys the structure and function of liver lobules

G. Occurs when restriction of blood flow through the liver increases pressure in the portal venous system

H. Removal of fluid from the peritoneal cavity

I. Fluid in the peritoneal cavity

J. Phase of hepatitis characterized by jaundice

## LEARNING OUTCOMES

1. Identify risk factors for pancreatitis.
2. Define *biliary colic*.
3. Describe foods to avoid in cholelithiasis.
4. Describe *hepatitis*.
5. List several reasons jaundice develops.
6. Identify people who should be vaccinated for hepatitis B.
7. Describe the pathophysiology of cirrhosis.
8. Identify diagnostic testing for cirrhosis.
9. Discuss manifestations of pancreatitis.
10. Describe lab tests for pancreatic disorders.

## APPLY WHAT YOU LEARNED

You are planning the discharge for Mr. W, who has been diagnosed with alcohol-induced cirrhosis. His medications are Aldactone, Riopan, lactulose, and a fluid restriction of 1,500 mL/day. He will return home, where he lives with his wife of 28 years. He has two children who are grown and live out of state.

1. What nursing interventions will be implemented?
2. What discharge instructions will the nurse review with the wife?
3. Identify nursing diagnoses for this patient.

## MULTIPLE CHOICE

Circle the answer that best completes the following statements.

1. You are discussing the various forms of hepatitis with the nursing instructor. She asks you which viral hepatitis is transmitted only by blood. Your response should be:
   A. G.
   B. E.
   C. D.
   D. C.

2. Which prescription would the nurse anticipate for a patient who has been diagnosed with cirrhosis of the liver?
   A. Lactulose
   B. Acetaminophen
   C. Ibuprofen
   D. Demerol

3. As a result of a patient's positive HIDA scan, the nurse expects his immediate treatment to include:
   A. high-protein diet.
   B. low-protein diet.
   C. high-fat diet.
   D. low-fat diet.

4. A patient has been diagnosed with acute pancreatitis. Which of the following complications should be anticipated by the nurse?
   A. Hypertension
   B. Flank bruising
   C. Hypoglycemia
   D. Fever

5. Mr. Blue, 48 years old, is diagnosed with cirrhosis of the liver. Which intervention should the nurse plan to include in the patient's skin care?
   A. Rub the skin briskly to aid in the drying process.
   B. Turn the patient every 20 minutes.
   C. Use hot water when bathing.
   D. Avoid soap for bathing.

6. You are preparing a patient for a paracentesis. Which of the following best explains the procedure?

    A. Fluid is removed from the retroperitoneal cavity.

    B. A long needle is inserted into the retroperitoneal cavity.

    C. A needle is inserted into the peritoneal cavity, and fluid is withdrawn.

    D. Fluid is removed from the thoracic cavity via a long needle.

7. The nurse is reviewing the lab results for a patient with acute pancreatitis. Which of the following would verify that this diagnosis is correct?

    A. Serum amylase 184 U/L

    B. Serum lipase 10 U/L

    C. Serum calcium 12 mg/dL

    D. WBC 5,500

8. A patient is receiving spironolactone for the treatment of cirrhosis. Which of the following statements, if made by the patient, would indicate that he understands the medication teaching?

    A. "I'm going to report any diarrhea to my doctor."

    B. "I should take this medication in the morning."

    C. "If I have any ringing in the ears, I'll call you."

    D. "I'll weigh myself every other day."

9. A patient returns from surgery with a T-tube. Which of the following interventions would NOT be appropriate for this patient?

    A. Place in Fowler's position.

    B. Keep the T-tube clamped.

    C. Monitor the color and consistency of drainage.

    D. Assess the skin for bile leakage.

10. When assessing a patient in the preicteric phase of acute viral hepatitis, the nurse would expect to identify which of these symptoms?

    A. Pruritus

    B. Clay-colored stools

    C. Flu-like symptoms

    D. Increased energy

11. A patient with acute hepatitis is experiencing anorexia and nausea. These signs would substantiate a nursing diagnosis of:

    A. Self-Care Deficit.

    B. Activity Intolerance.

    C. Risk for Infection.

    D. Altered Nutrition: Less Than Body Requirements.

12. Which of these events, if present in a patient's history, is most likely related to the development of hepatitis?

    A. Injection drug user

    B. Recent travel to Florida

    C. Viral infection of the upper airway

    D. History of flu vaccine

13. You are assisting in a liver biopsy. If all of the following are postprocedure nursing interventions, which should be your highest priority?

    A. Position the patient on his or her right side.

    B. Keep NPO for 2 hours.

    C. Frequently assess the site.

    D. Apply direct pressure after the needle is removed.

14. The nurse is teaching a patient about the importance of bleeding precautions. Which of the following should NOT be included in the care plan?

    A. Avoid blowing nose.

    B. Use a medium–hard toothbrush.

    C. Assess for purpura.

    D. Avoid injections.

15. Lactulose is frequently used in the treatment of hepatic encephalopathy. The purpose of this medication is to:

    A. inhibit ammonia absorption from the bowel.

    B. destroy intestinal bacteria.

    C. reduce ascites.

    D. reduce peristalsis.

# CHAPTER 28 ▶ The Urinary System and Assessment

## KEY TERMS

Match each term with its appropriate definition.

1. Glomeruli
2. Nephrons
3. Urinalysis
4. Renal arteriogram
5. Glomerular filtration rate
6. Pyuria
7. Nocturia
8. Dysuria
9. Voiding studies
10. Hematuria

A. Painful urination
B. Done to visualize and evaluate renal blood vessels and blood flow through the kidneys
C. Functional units of the kidney
D. Small clusters of capillaries
E. Rate at which blood is filtered in the glomeruli
F. Key part of the diagnostic evaluation of the urinary system
G. Urinating more than one time at night
H. Cloudy, foul-smelling urine
I. Used to evaluate voiding and lower urinary tract function, urinary retention, and urinary incontinence
J. Blood in the urine

## LEARNING OUTCOMES

1. What is the purpose of nephrons?
2. Describe the function of the ureters.
3. Describe the glomerular filtration process.
4. Identify the normal glomerular filtration rate.
5. Discuss the differences between dysuria, nocturia, and hematuria.
6. Identify laboratory tests commonly used to evaluate renal function.
7. Define *uroflowmetry*.
8. Describe the 24-hour urine specimen process.
9. Identify teaching points regarding a cystoscopy.
10. Describe components involved in urine studies.

## APPLY WHAT YOU LEARNED

A newly admitted male patient is being tested because of complaints related to pain upon urination. The patient is offering vague descriptions of his symptoms. The physician has ordered blood work and a 24-hour urine test along with some imaging studies.

1. Describe the procedure involved in a 24-hour urine specimen collection.
2. What imaging studies will be done for this patient?
3. What is the physician looking for in the blood work related to kidney function?

## MULTIPLE CHOICE

Circle the answer that best completes the following statements.

1. Your patient has been ordered to have a postvoid residual catheterization. Which of the following statements made by the patient indicates understanding of the procedure?
   - A. "I will call you after I have gone to the bathroom and urinated."
   - B. "I will be sure to flush the toilet after I have voided."
   - C. "As soon as I void, the nurse will catheterize me."
   - D. "The nurse will leave the catheter in place after the procedure."

2. When obtaining a health history from Katie about her urinary status, the nurse asks all of the following questions EXCEPT:
   - A. "Are you going to the bathroom frequently?"
   - B. "Have you noticed blood in your urine?"
   - C. "Do you have discharge from your vagina after intercourse?"
   - D. "What is your fluid intake during the day?"

3. In a renal clearance, there are two substances found in the blood that are routinely used to evaluate renal function. The effective indicators of renal function are:
   - A. blood urea and GFR.
   - B. BUN and serum creatinine.
   - C. GFR and BUN.
   - D. uric acid levels and creatinine.

4. You are asked to obtain a sterile urine sample from an older patient with dementia. The first action should be to:
   - A. cleanse the perineal area.
   - B. label the container.
   - C. place the patient in the dorsal recumbent position.
   - D. obtain all the supplies needed.

5. A 24-hour urine test is also known as a:
   - A. blood urea nitrogen test.
   - B. GFR.
   - C. creatinine clearance test.
   - D. KUB.

6. The physician has ordered a 24-hour urine test for a patient with renal disease. The test is to begin at 6 A.M. At what time should the patient empty his bladder and discard the urine?

   A. 5 A.M.

   B. 5:30 A.M.

   C. 6 A.M.

   D. The patient does not discard any urine.

7. Nursing care for the patient to evaluate urinary retention and incontinence includes all of the following EXCEPT:

   A. administering pain medications.

   B. using an uroflowmeter.

   C. obtaining a specimen.

   D. measuring urine output.

8. A urinalysis has just been received on the unit for Mr. Kattes. The nurse is aware that a normal urinalysis should not have:

   A. ketones—negative.

   B. protein—10 mg/dL.

   C. WBC—3 to 4/LPF.

   D. glucose—negative.

9. Ultrasound examination of the bladder or kidneys is a noninvasive examination that requires:

   A. the patient to ingest dye to see the organs.

   B. an empty stomach.

   C. no preparation of the patient.

   D. a full bladder.

10. When teaching a patient about a renal scan, the nurse informs her that she must increase fluid intake:

    A. before and after the scan.

    B. 4 hours before the scan.

    C. after the scan only.

    D. before the scan only.

11. The functional unit of the kidney is known as the:

    A. ureter.

    B. nephron.

    C. urethra.

    D. glomerulus.

12. The nurse understands the normal GFR in adults is:

    A. 50 to 75 mL/min.

    B. 100 to 200 mL/min.

    C. 120 to 125 mL/min.

    D. 10 to 15 mL/min.

13. Foul-smelling urine with a cloudy appearance is known as:
    A. nocturia.
    B. hematuria.
    C. dysuria.
    D. pyuria.

14. Direct visualization of the urethra and bladder using an endoscope is known as:
    A. cystoscopy.
    B. renal scan.
    C. ultrasound.
    D. computed tomography.

15. Urine is concentrated in which structure of the kidney?
    A. Loop of Henle
    B. Ureter
    C. Urethra
    D. Bladder

# CHAPTER 29 ▶ Caring for Patients With Kidney and Urinary Tract Disorders

## KEY TERMS

Match each term with its appropriate definition.

1. Dialysis
2. Kidney failure
3. Urgency
4. Hematuria
5. Cystitis
6. Pyelonephritis
7. Glomerulonephritis
8. Azotemia
9. Dialysate
10. Urolithiasis

A. Condition in which the kidneys are unable to remove accumulated waste products from the blood
B. An inflammatory disorder affecting the renal pelvis
C. Used to remove excess fluid and waste products in renal failure
D. Increased blood levels of nitrogenous wastes, including urea and creatinine
E. Dialysis solution
F. The most common cause of obstructed urine flow
G. Sudden, compelling need to urinate
H. Blood in the urine
I. The most common UTI
J. May be an acute or a chronic disorder

## LEARNING OUTCOMES

1. Define *urinary incontinence*.
2. Identify the types of urinary incontinence.
3. Identify manifestations of urinary tract infections in older adults.
4. Define *azotemia*.
5. Describe manifestations of urinary stones.
6. Identify foods that are high in purines.
7. Describe nursing diagnoses related to bladder cancer.
8. Discuss some problems patients may have related to dialysis.
9. Describe *renal failure*.
10. Discuss implementations of nursing care for excess fluid volume.

# APPLY WHAT YOU LEARNED

You are caring for a 72-year-old female with renal failure. The physician has ordered dialysis. The patient will be having an arteriovenous fistula placed in the morning. She has a strong support system with many family members, including her spouse. Her psychosocial assessment reveals a poor understanding of her condition.

1. How would the nurse describe renal failure to this patient and her family to ensure understanding?
2. Describe the process of dialysis.
3. What are some nursing diagnoses that apply to this patient?

# MULTIPLE CHOICE

Circle the answer that best completes the following statements.

1. Which of the following is the most important point to remember when performing a urinary catheterization?
   A. Assess the amount and color of the initial drainage.
   B. Provide perineal care before performing the procedure.
   C. Use sterile technique when inserting the catheter.
   D. Do not drain more than 800 mL of urine from the bladder.

2. A middle-aged female patient is having a minor problem with stress incontinence. Which of the following nursing interventions would NOT be included in the nursing care plan?
   A. Monitor intake and output.
   B. Teach Kegel exercises.
   C. Try to hold the urine as long as possible before going to the bathroom.
   D. Limit beverages after the evening meal.

3. The nurse is teaching a young female how to decrease the risk for a UTI. If all of the following are true, which statement should have the highest priority?
   A. Do not use bubble bath.
   B. Wipe from front to back.
   C. Do not use a diaphragm for birth control.
   D. Empty the bladder at least every 2 hours.

4. A patient asks the nurse about complementary therapies for preventing a UTI. Which of the following fruits would be recommended for this patient?
   A. Blueberries
   B. Grape juice
   C. Oranges
   D. Pineapple

5. A 28-year-old patient has been admitted to the orthopedic floor after sustaining multiple rib fractures in a motorcycle crash. The physician should be notified if the patient develops:
   A. bruising on the chest wall.
   B. a fever of 100 degrees.
   C. oliguria.
   D. an increased appetite.

6. A patient receiving Gantrisin for a UTI developed a rash several hours after taking the first dose. The nurse's best response to this development is:

   **A.** "The rash is normal. It will go away in a few days."

   **B.** "You didn't tell me that you were allergic to a sulfa drug!"

   **C.** "Don't take any more of the medication. I will notify the doctor."

   **D.** "I should have looked at your chart before I gave you the mediation."

7. Which of the following should be included in the teaching plan for a patient with an order for Pyridium?

   **A.** Take the medication for at least 3 days.

   **B.** Take the drug on an empty stomach.

   **C.** The medication will clear up the infection in 1 week.

   **D.** Wear a peripad to protect your underwear.

8. A patient has been ordered a low-purine diet. The dietary department calls you to confirm the choices made on the menu. You realize that your patient needs further teaching because he ordered:

   **A.** crab.

   **B.** tuna.

   **C.** fried trout.

   **D.** liver.

9. Which symptom is the patient with bladder cancer most likely to exhibit?

   **A.** Painless hematuria

   **B.** Urinary frequency

   **C.** Dysuria

   **D.** Back pain

10. A patient has been admitted for major trauma to the pelvis. The physician tells you that the patient is hypovolemic and orders an IV NS at 150 mL/hr. Based on this information, you should monitor closely for signs of:

    **A.** acute renal failure.

    **B.** spontaneous pneumothorax.

    **C.** chronic renal failure.

    **D.** urolithiasis.

11. Which type of incontinence is brought on by sneezing, laughing, or lifting?

    **A.** Stress

    **B.** Urge

    **C.** Overflow

    **D.** Reflex

12. The nurse understands what about incontinence?

    **A.** It is a normal part of the aging process.

    **B.** All people over 65 have some form of it.

    **C.** It is not a normal part of the aging process.

    **D.** It affects only people over 80.

13. The condition occurring when trauma interferes with the normal mechanisms of bladder emptying is known as:

   A. neurogenic bladder.

   B. spastic bladder.

   C. benign prostatic hypertrophy.

   D. cystitis.

14. Which of the following is NOT a manifestation of cystitis?

   A. Dysuria

   B. Hematuria

   C. Incontinence

   D. Frequency

15. A removal of the entire urinary bladder and surrounding tissues is known as:

   A. ileal conduit.

   B. radical cystectomy.

   C. partial cystectomy.

   D. cutaneous ureterostomy.

# CHAPTER 30

## The Reproductive System and Assessment

### KEY TERMS

Match each term with its appropriate definition.

1. Mammography
2. Colposcopy
3. Follicle-stimulating hormone
4. Contraception
5. Androgens
6. Lithotomy position
7. Ejaculation
8. Libido
9. Spermatogenesis
10. Estrogens

A. Male sex hormones

B. Used to examine tissues of the vagina and cervix using a brightly lighted microscope

C. Steroid hormones essential to the development and maintenance of female secondary sex characteristics

D. Produced by the anterior pituitary gland; levels are measured to evaluate menstrual disorders, amenorrhea, or infertility

E. Sperm production

F. Sexual desire

G. Supine position with knees flexed and separated

H. Expulsion of seminal fluid

I. Radiologic procedure used to screen for breast cancer in women who have no symptoms

J. Avoidance of pregnancy while maintaining the ability to have heterosexual sexual intercourse

### LEARNING OUTCOMES

1. Identify the structures of the male reproductive system.
2. Identify the internal structures of the female reproductive system.
3. List three hormones the ovaries produce.
4. Describe the purpose of mammography.
5. Describe the pelvic ultrasound.
6. Discuss transrectal ultrasonography.
7. Describe the prostate gland.
8. Describe the phases of the ovarian cycle.
9. Describe spermatogenesis.
10. Describe seminal fluid.

## APPLY WHAT YOU LEARNED

An adolescent presented in the clinic with the onset of her first period. The student nurse is currently studying reproduction and knows that this is often a sensitive subject for teen girls to discuss. The patient's mother is not with her, and she does not know that this is the beginning of a cycle into womanhood.

1. Explain the menstrual cycle.
2. How would the nurse comfort this patient and ensure her dignity?

## MULTIPLE CHOICE

Circle the answer that best completes the following statements.

1. While palpating the inguinal and groin areas of her male patient, the nurse knows she is checking for a possible:
   A. STI.
   B. BPH.
   C. bulges.
   D. testicular injury.

2. The nurse knows that when palpating the breast for discharge, the nipples must be:
   A. pinched.
   B. rolled.
   C. pulled.
   D. compressed.

3. What is the correct position for a female while her vagina is being assessed?
   A. Supine
   B. Lithotomy
   C. Semi-Fowler's
   D. Knees to chest

4. Tumors that are too small to be detected by clinical breast exam or self-breast exam can be identified by:
   A. mammography.
   B. x-ray.
   C. CT scan.
   D. MRI.

5. When teaching a patient about laparoscopy, the nurse must remember to tell the patient that the night before the exam she must:
   A. eat.
   B. keep her bladder full.
   C. douche.
   D. discuss the treatment methods with her spouse.

6. Instruct the patient having mammography that 5 to 7 days before the exam she must avoid caffeine and:

   A. carbonated drinks.

   B. blueberries.

   C. purines.

   D. methylxanthines.

7. Colposcopy can identify early premalignant changes in cervical tissue and is performed when abnormal results are found on:

   A. CT.

   B. endoscopy.

   C. Pap smear.

   D. MRI.

8. In men, the urethra and penis both serve as organs for urine elimination and ejaculation of:

   A. sperm.

   B. bacteria.

   C. oocytes.

   D. enzymes.

9. Bill has been complaining of a loss in libido. His serum testosterone level is 500 ng/dL. Normal serum levels are:

   A. 650 to 2,000 ng/dL.

   B. 300 to 1,000 ng/dL.

   C. 150 to 500 ng/dL.

   D. 1 to 50 ng/dL.

10. What could be another possible problem with Bill's loss of libido?

    A. Drinking

    B. Medications

    C. Mental concerns

    D. All of the above

11. The term used to describe male sex hormones is:

    A. scrotum.

    B. testes.

    C. estrogens.

    D. androgens.

12. The outer layer of the uterine wall is known as:

    A. perimetrium.

    B. myometrium.

    C. endometrium.

    D. endocervical.

13. The nurse knows that the vaginal mucus is bacteriostatic and:

   A. alkaline.

   B. acidic.

   C. phosphoric.

   D. calciumated.

14. The lab test done to evaluate the function of the testes and ovaries is:

   A. serum estradiol.

   B. progesterone.

   C. serum testosterone.

   D. follicle-stimulating hormone.

15. CA125 is a marker used to detect which cancer?

   A. Ovarian

   B. Breast

   C. Testicular

   D. Uterine

# CHAPTER 31 ▶ *Caring for Male Patients With Reproductive System Disorders*

## KEY TERMS

Match each term with its appropriate definition.

1. Benign prostatic hyperplasia
2. Vasectomy
3. Orchiectomy
4. Erectile dysfunction
5. Infertility
6. Gynecomastia
7. Transurethral resection of the prostate
8. Cryptorchidism
9. Impotence
10. Prostatectomy

A. A sterilization procedure in which a portion of the spermatic cord is removed

B. Failure of one or both testes to descend through the inguinal ring into the scrotum

C. Also called impotence

D. Enlargement of the prostate gland

E. Removal of the testes

F. Surgical removal of the prostate gland

G. Inability to conceive a child during a year or more of unprotected intercourse

H. Obstructing prostate tissue is removed using a wire loop inserted through the urethra

I. Inability to attain and maintain an erection that allows satisfactory sexual intercourse

J. Breast enlargement

## LEARNING OUTCOMES

1. Describe the pathophysiology of BPH.
2. Identify manifestations of prostate cancer.
3. Describe diagnostic testing regarding the prostate.
4. List instances in which radiation might be used in the context of male reproductive system disorders.
5. Describe the three approaches to a prostatectomy.
6. Identify nursing diagnoses related to prostate dysfunction.
7. Define *testicular torsion*.
8. What is an important teaching point for the patient with cryptorchidism?
9. Discuss testicular cancer.
10. List several diagnostic tests related to erectile dysfunction.

## APPLY WHAT YOU LEARNED

A 61-year-old male patient presents to your clinic with complaints of urgency regarding urination. During the physical exam, the physician palpates a hard nodule on the prostate gland. Upon further assessment, the patient tells the physician that he has been getting up three or four times a night to use the bathroom and not much urine comes out when he tries.

1. What diagnostic testing would the nurse expect the physician to order to follow up on the nodule?
2. Would this patient be a candidate for a surgical procedure? If so, which one?
3. Describe some teaching that the nurse would do with the patient and his partner.

## MULTIPLE CHOICE

Circle the answer that best completes the following statements.

1. The nurse has instructed a male patient in testicular self-examination. Further teaching is required when the patient says:
   A. "The day I do the exam should be the same day each month."
   B. "It is good to perform the exam in the shower."
   C. "My testicles should feel smooth and walnut sized."
   D. "I will check myself before I have sexual intercourse."

2. You are bathing a male patient and notice that he is not circumcised. You pull back the foreskin. After you have cleansed the penis, which of the following must be done?
   A. Have the patient empty his bladder.
   B. Replace the foreskin.
   C. Clean the anal area.
   D. Document the bath on the nursing notes.

3. Which of the following patients has an increased risk of developing priapism?
   A. 22-year-old male with spinal cord trauma
   B. 35-year-old male with testicular injury
   C. 62-year-old male with BPH
   D. 84-year-old male with impotence

4. The nursing assistant reports that Mr. Peterson has a sore on his penis. He denies any pain. Your best response should be to say:
   A. "Okay, just be sure and wash him real well."
   B. "I'll be there in a few minutes to take a look at the sore."
   C. "It's probably nothing. Just document it in the nurse's notes."
   D. "It's probably cancer. I'll let the doctor know right away."

5. A patient has been diagnosed with erectile dysfunction. If all of the following are appropriate nursing interventions, which should have the highest priority?
   A. Actively listen to your patient's concerns.
   B. Teach the patient about the condition.
   C. Explain to the patient the importance of pelvic floor exercises.
   D. Discuss the treatment methods.

6. When preparing a patient for a transrectal ultrasound-guided biopsy of the prostate, the teaching plan should include which of these instructions?

    A. The patient will be fully unconscious during the procedure.

    B. An informed consent is not necessary.

    C. Hematuria and bloody streaks are expected several days after the procedure.

    D. Advise the patient to continue on his daily dose of aspirin.

7. Which of these statements, if made by the patient diagnosed with prostate cancer, would support a nursing diagnosis of Deficient Knowledge?

    A. "There isn't much hope for me, is there?"

    B. "My doctor said I might have some impotence problems after my surgery."

    C. "The hormone therapy won't cure my cancer."

    D. "If I don't get treated, my cancer might go to my lungs."

8. A patient is being treated for prostatitis. The nurse should include which of the following diagnoses in the care plan?

    A. Ineffective Protection related to depressed immune system

    B. Fear related to possible death

    C. Activity Intolerance related to fatigue

    D. Disturbed Body Image related to physical changes

9. The nurse is explaining various approaches to a prostatectomy. She would be correct in stating that a suprapubic prostatectomy is done through an:

    A. incision between the scrotum and the anus.

    B. abdominal incision into the bladder.

    C. abdominal incision with the bladder remaining intact.

    D. insertion of a Foley catheter.

10. A patient is receiving Viagra. The nurse should plan to observe for side effects, which include:

    A. phimosis.

    B. hypertension.

    C. hypokalemia.

    D. hypotension.

11. Which of these measures should be included in the care plan for a patient who is recovering from a TURP?

    A. Use clean technique when handling the drainage system.

    B. Frequently assess catheter patency.

    C. Obtain intake and output every 24 hours.

    D. Maintain the CBI to keep the output cherry red.

12. A patient presents with complaints that he has no sexual desire. You anticipate that the physician may order a:

    A. psychologic consult.

    B. testosterone level.

    C. routine urinalysis.

    D. PSA.

13. A patient asks you what complementary therapies are available for BPH. Your best response should be:

   A. "I can't talk about other treatments, that's the doctor's job."

   B. "Yoga can help you to relax."

   C. "Saw palmetto grass has been known to reduce the symptoms."

   D. "Flomax helps to relax the smooth muscle."

14. Which nursing intervention would be the most appropriate to meet the expected outcome of "patient will wake up less frequently during the night" for a patient who has BPH?

   A. Advise patient to restrict alcohol intake.

   B. Provide information about his condition.

   C. Determine his level of anxiety.

   D. Provide pain measures during the day.

15. The patient who is at the highest risk for orchitis is the:

   A. 10-year-old male with measles.

   B. 38-year-old male with HIV.

   C. 42-year-old male with prostate cancer.

   D. 48-year-old male with mumps.

# CHAPTER 32

# Caring for Female Patients With Reproductive System Disorders

## KEY TERMS

Match each term with its appropriate definition.

1. Mastectomy
2. Dyspareunia
3. PMS
4. Dysmenorrhea
5. DUB
6. Hysterectomy
7. Salpingo-oophorectomy
8. Menopause
9. Amenorrhea
10. Infertility

A. Pain associated with menstruation

B. Absence of menstruation

C. Removal of the breast

D. Pain during sexual intercourse

E. Vaginal bleeding that is abnormal in amount, duration, or time of occurrence

F. A symptom complex of irritability, depression, edema, and breast tenderness preceding menses

G. Period during which menstruation permanently ceases

H. Removal of the uterus

I. Inability to get pregnant with unprotected intercourse for at least 1 year

J. Removal of both fallopian tubes and ovaries

## LEARNING OUTCOMES

1. List several complementary therapies for menopause.
2. Describe hormone replacement therapy.
3. Discuss premenstrual syndrome.
4. Define *hysterectomy*.
5. Describe endometriosis.
6. Identify diagnostic testing related to ovarian cysts.
7. Define *vaginitis*.
8. Describe pelvic inflammatory disease.
9. Discuss cervical cancer.
10. Define *uterine prolapse*.

## APPLY WHAT YOU LEARNED

A 35-year-old female comes into the emergency department with complaints of nipple discharge, breast pain, and a persistent skin rash near the nipple. She states it started about a week ago, and she was going to wait to see if it cleared up on its own. She is not due for her yearly gynecological exam and has not had a mammogram before. She states that three of her aunts on her mother's side have had breast cancer.

1.  What risk factors does this patient have that would make the nurse suspect breast cancer?
2.  What diagnostic testing is done to confirm breast cancer?
3.  Identify nursing diagnoses related to this patient.
4.  Describe the grieving process regarding this situation.

## MULTIPLE CHOICE

Circle the answer that best completes the following statements.

1.  The nurse is teaching a group of middle school girls the signs of breast cancer. Which of the following would she not include in the lecture?
    A.  Nipple discharge
    B.  Unusual lump in the axilla
    C.  Small, hard, painless lump in the breast
    D.  Brown area around the nipple

2.  A patient who is scheduled for a breast biopsy may need further instruction if she says:
    A.  "The doctor will numb my breast."
    B.  "I will be sure to sit up straight so the best sample can be obtained."
    C.  "Some of my breast tissue will be removed using a needle."
    D.  "I can use ice packs if I feel discomfort."

3.  You are explaining to your patient why, following pelvic surgery, she should stop smoking. The best explanation would be:
    A.  "Because it is bad for your health."
    B.  "To avoid complications related to urinary incontinence."
    C.  "Because stopping will help with the grieving process."
    D.  "To try to avoid deep venous thrombosis and pulmonary embolism."

4.  A 52-year-old patient is upset about the onset of menopause. She asks the nurse how she can cope with the symptoms. The best response should be:
    A.  "Avoid drinking alcohol and caffeine."
    B.  "Everyone has to go through these changes."
    C.  "Splash your face with warm water to relax your muscles."
    D.  "Keep the room warm, especially at night."

5.  The nurse knows which patient is most at risk for PID?
    A.  The 12-year-old girl who is not yet menstruating
    B.  The 43-year-old-woman who uses condoms for birth control
    C.  The 18-year-old sexually active woman
    D.  The 64-year-old woman whose husband died a year ago

6. A patient presents to the emergency department with a temperature of 103°F and vomiting. Your assessment reveals hypotension and peeling skin on her palms and feet. There is a foul-smelling discharge from her vagina. The patient states that she is on her menses and has a tampon in place. Your next action would be to:

    A. place the patient in the lithotomy position.

    B. ask the patient to remove the tampon.

    C. ask the patient if she is pregnant.

    D. remove the tampon.

7. The nurse recognizes that which factor in the patient's history is the most important etiological factor in developing cervical cancer?

    A. Intercourse using a latex condom

    B. Monogamous relationship

    C. Infection with HPV

    D. Poor hygiene

8. Tamoxifen is most often used for the patient with breast cancer because it:

    A. inhibits growth of the tumor by blocking estrogen receptor sites.

    B. replaces lost estrogen needed for cancer protection.

    C. reduces the risk of endometrial cancer.

    D. decreases the spread of breast cancer.

9. A patient tells the nurse that she has a fishy-smelling, "milklike" discharge from her vagina. The nurse suspects that this patient has:

    A. atrophic vaginitis.

    B. candidiasis.

    C. trichomoniasis.

    D. simple vaginitis.

10. Which of the following patients is most likely to develop breast cancer in her lifetime?

    A. A patient with a familial history of colon cancer

    B. A patient who started her menstrual period at 14 years of age

    C. A patient who had multiple chest x-rays before she was 30 years old

    D. A patient who had her first child at the age of 22

11. Upon admission to the medical floor, the nurse should give highest priority to meeting which need of a patient diagnosed with PID?

    A. Information related to the prevention of PID

    B. Pain control

    C. Insertion of a Foley catheter

    D. Ordering daily meals

12. A postmastectomy patient refuses to do arm exercises because of the presence of a JP drain. The nurse should tell the patient:

    A. "It's ok. You can wait until you are ready."

    B. "Remember that it is important to begin exercising now to restore full mobility."

    C. "You are right. You need to wait until your stitches are removed."

    D. "Please do your exercises now and remember to use aseptic technique."

13. In preparing a care plan for a patient diagnosed with dysfunctional uterine bleeding, it is most important for the nurse to include a goal that addresses the need for:

    **A.** sexual function concerns.

    **B.** increased compliance with the medication regime.

    **C.** information on how to promote conception.

    **D.** wound care management.

14. A patient has been told that abnormal cells were seen in her initial Pap test. The next action taken by the nurse should be to:

    **A.** prepare the patient for a hysterectomy.

    **B.** ask the patient if she has any questions about the repeat Pap test.

    **C.** begin an IV of NS in preparation for cauterization of the abnormal cells.

    **D.** ask the patient to sign another consent form.

15. The physician suspects that a patient has DUB. Which of the following lab tests would NOT be ordered to confirm the diagnosis?

    **A.** PSA

    **B.** CBC

    **C.** Pap smear

    **D.** Thyroid function tests

# CHAPTER 33 ▶ Caring for Patients With Sexually Transmitted Infections

## KEY TERMS

Match each term with its appropriate definition.

1. Abstinence
2. Vulva
3. Infertility
4. Syphilis
5. Prodromal symptoms
6. Mutual monogamy
7. Female condom
8. Chancre
9. Vesicles
10. Sexually transmitted infection

A. Painless ulcer
B. Lubricated polyurethane sheath inserted into the vagina
C. Inability to conceive or initiate pregnancy
D. Having sex with a partner who has sex only with you
E. Caused by a spirochete
F. Blisters
G. Voluntarily refraining from sexual intercourse
H. Transmitted by sexual contact, including vaginal, oral, and anal intercourse
I. Perineal area outside the vagina
J. Warning signals of an impending outbreak

## LEARNING OUTCOMES

1. Discuss who is at risk for STIs.
2. Identify risk factors for STIs.
3. Describe chlamydia.
4. Describe the presentation of gonorrhea.
5. Identify nursing diagnoses related to STIs.
6. Discuss the prevention of STIs.
7. Define *genital herpes.*
8. Describe syphilis.
9. Describe manifestations of trichomoniasis.
10. Identify the STIs that are reportable to state and federal agencies.

# APPLY WHAT YOU LEARNED

The student nurse is presenting sexual education information to the local high school with the rest of his nursing class. The class has numerous handouts, posters, quizzes, and self-assessment tests for the teens. The student nurse feels well prepared and nervous at the same time due to the sensitive nature of the topic.

1. What interventions could the student nurse use to feel at ease and put the teens at ease?
2. What subjective and objective assessment data related to STIs will the student nurse discuss with the teens?
3. Which risk factors will the student nurse elaborate on during the discussion with the teens?

# MULTIPLE CHOICE

Circle the answer that best completes the following statements.

1. Ms. Doyle is examined by the nurse practitioner. The diagnosis is chlamydia. Which of the following interventions would best meet the need for preventing transmission of the organism?
   A. Encourage her partner to get medical attention.
   B. Recommend abstinence while the lesions are healing.
   C. Provide social and emotional support.
   D. Explain the life cycle of chlamydia.

2. A nurse is teaching a sex education class to a group of high school students. To gain a better understanding of their level of knowledge, the nurse asks the students to say the name of the most common reportable communicable disease in the United States. The correct response is:
   A. syphilis.
   B. chlamydia.
   C. gonorrhea.
   D. genital herpes.

3. A patient admits that he forgets to take the medication prescribed for his gonorrhea. The most effective method to overcome this noncompliance would be to:
   A. call him on the telephone as a reminder.
   B. make an appointment with his case worker.
   C. provide extensive education about his infection.
   D. administer a single dose of medication as ordered.

4. A young man is seen at the emergency department for profuse and purulent urethral discharge. It is important that the nurse gather information related to:
   A. previous infections.
   B. all sexual contacts.
   C. a history of bladder infections.
   D. recent sexual contacts.

5. After assessing an 18-year-old patient, the nurse makes the diagnosis of Ineffective Health Maintenance. The nurse understands that further teaching is necessary because the patient has:

   A. a stable monogamous relationship with her boyfriend.

   B. never been tested for chlamydia.

   C. had annual Pap smears.

   D. multiple sex partners.

6. Mr. Black was diagnosed with gonorrhea and has been treated with ceftriaxone IM in a single injection plus azithromycin PO in a single dose. He is given a prescription for doxycycline to take at home. The nurse explains that this combination of antibiotics is prescribed to:

   A. treat any coexisting chlamydial infection.

   B. eliminate resistant strains of gonorrhea.

   C. prevent the development of resistant organisms.

   D. prevent reinfection.

7. Sally Hart has primary syphilis. While caring for her the nurse should:

   A. wear gloves when taking her vital signs.

   B. place the patient in isolation.

   C. assess the feet for the presence of blisters.

   D. discuss safer sex practices.

8. The nurse suspects that the patient does not understand the disease process of genital herpes when he says:

   A. "Once I finish taking my medication, my herpes will be cured."

   B. "I should abstain from having sex when the lesions are present."

   C. "Docosanol 10% cream can be applied to the lesions."

   D. "It would be a good idea to purchase some boxer shorts and wear them during the outbreak."

9. A young patient tells you that her girlfriend said that "a person would get cancer if they had the papilloma virus." Your best response should be:

   A. "Your girlfriend isn't your doctor."

   B. "There is a greater risk of cervical cancer for those infected with HPV."

   C. "I've never heard of that."

   D. "That idea is just a myth. Just ignore her."

10. A patient is being treated for chlamydia. The nurse knows that the teaching has been effective when the patient states:

    A. "One injection of penicillin will cure me."

    B. "Use of a spermicidal foam will protect me from further infections."

    C. "Even if I don't get treated, the chlamydia will eventually go away."

    D. "I need to tell my boyfriend so he can get treated."

11. A 24-year-old patient tells you that her boyfriend left her because she has genital warts. She says that he "thought they were disgusting." Based on this information, the nurse makes a diagnosis of:

   **A.** Ineffective Individual Coping.

   **B.** Anxiety.

   **C.** Risk for Infection.

   **D.** Disturbed Body Image.

12. You are collecting data from the chart of a patient, age 17, to assist in the development of the nursing care plan. You note that this patient has been pregnant three times. If all of the following are risk factors for contracting an STI, which should be given priority when talking with the patient?

   **A.** Use of oral contraceptives

   **B.** Adolescent sexual activity

   **C.** Multiple sex partners

   **D.** Unprotected sexual activity

13. The nurse is discussing discharge instructions with a patient who has the "clap." The most important point that should be emphasized is:

   **A.** take all of the prescribed medication.

   **B.** use a condom for sexual intercourse.

   **C.** encourage sexual partners to be treated.

   **D.** return for follow-up appointment.

14. The risk for contracting any STI is directly related to:

   **A.** the number of sexual partners.

   **B.** lifestyle.

   **C.** age.

   **D.** gender.

15. Which of the following must be reported to the public health department?

   **A.** Genital herpes

   **B.** Syphilis

   **C.** Chlamydia

   **D.** Trichomoniasis

# CHAPTER 34 ▶ *The Endocrine System and Assessment*

## KEY TERMS

Match each term with its appropriate definition.

1. Hyperglycemia
2. Hypoglycemia
3. Hormones
4. Exophthalmos
5. Iodine
6. Islets of Langerhans
7. Epinephrine
8. Glycogenolysis
9. Gluconeogenesis
10. Adrenal medulla

A. Necessary for proper functioning of the thyroid

B. Process of making new glucose

C. High blood glucose level

D. The body's chemical messengers

E. Forward protrusion of the eyeballs

F. Release insulin into the bloodstream

G. Low blood glucose level

H. A counterregulatory hormone

I. Produces hormones known as catecholamines

J. Processes of converting glycogen into glucose in the liver and muscles

## LEARNING OUTCOMES

1. Describe the purpose of the endocrine system.
2. Identify the lab tests ordered to diagnose an endocrine disorder.
3. Describe how an MRI is used as a diagnostic tool.
4. Discuss the function of the thyroid gland.
5. Describe the functions of the hypothalamus.
6. Explain the purpose of the pancreas.
7. Identify the purpose of insulin.
8. Describe exophthalmos.
9. Discuss the 2-hour oral glucose tolerance test.
10. Explain the purpose of the adrenal cortex.

## APPLY WHAT YOU LEARNED

A nursing student is learning about the importance of the endocrine system, and she realizes that hormones and insulin regulate many parts of the body. While at a clinical rotation, the student is asked to explain the structure and function of the endocrine system.

1. What hormones would she say are associated with the anterior pituitary?
2. How would she explain the functions of these hormones?

## MULTIPLE CHOICE

Circle the answer that best completes the following statements.

1. The nurse is preparing a poster for a health fair and knows that which of the following should be presented as functions of the thyroid gland?
   A. Stimulates breast milk production, controls pigmentation of the skin
   B. Increases metabolic rate, lowers serum calcium levels
   C. Regulates blood volume and electrolytes
   D. Promotes water retention by kidneys, promotes uterine contraction

2. The nurse is preparing a patient for her MRI. Which of the following is an important step to take in this preparation?
   A. To collect a fresh urine sample
   B. To assess for any metallic implants such as pacemakers
   C. To ask about allergies to iodine and seafood
   D. To make sure the patient has fasted for at least 8 hours

3. Mrs. Leopold presents with a temperature of 99°F, malaise, and says, "I feel tired all the time." Subsequent labs reveal a $T_4$ of 0.5 mcg/dL. You suspect that Mrs. Leopold will be diagnosed with:
   A. Cushing syndrome.
   B. severe bronchitis.
   C. hypothyroidism.
   D. sepsis.

4. Which of the following is NOT part of the endocrine system?
   A. Liver
   B. Anterior pituitary
   C. Gonads
   D. Pancreas

5. The nurse who is explaining the concept of negative feedback as it relates to the endocrine system can best compare the process to:
   A. the way a small child learns to tie his shows.
   B. the change of seasons.
   C. Pavlovian fear conditioning.
   D. the way the thermostat in a house regulates temperature.

6. The nurse understands that the pituitary gland is located:

    A. on top of the kidneys.

    B. in the skull, beneath the hypothalamus.

    C. to the side of the trachea.

    D. on the posterior lobes of the thyroid gland.

7. What is the primary function of insulin?

    A. To produce glucagon

    B. To constrict blood vessels

    C. To regulate blood glucose levels

    D. To maintain normal salt and water balance

8. The nurse understands that assessment of endocrine function can be difficult because:

    A. definitions of normal blood glucose levels vary in clinical practice, depending on the laboratory that performs the assay.

    B. hormones affect all body tissues and organs, so manifestations of endocrine dysfunction are often nonspecific.

    C. the nurse must determine whether the patient has become more sensitive to heat or cold.

    D. a health assessment interview to identify problems with the endocrine system may be part of a general health screening.

9. A patient who has recently developed exophthalmos tells you that she has stopped dating. She tells you that she thought her eyes would return to "normal" after her diagnosis of Graves disease. A primary nursing diagnosis would be:

    A. Ineffective Health Maintenance

    B. Disturbed Personal Identity

    C. Deficient Knowledge

    D. Risk for Situational Low Self-Esteem

10. When assessing an older adult patient, the nurse knows it is important to remember that:

    A. lung sounds do not need to be assessed as part of an older adult's endocrine assessment.

    B. the older adult may get fatigued more quickly, so the nurse needs to perform a fast assessment.

    C. the physician will likely order an MRI because of the special needs of the older adult patient.

    D. there is an unclear relationship between aging and endocrine function.

11. What is the first step of physically assessing a patient's endocrine function?

    A. Assess the patient's general appearance and document vital signs, height, and weight.

    B. Inspect for gynecomastia.

    C. Palpate hands and feet for edema.

    D. Auscultate lungs for adventitious sounds.

12. When collecting data on a patient suspected of having an endocrine disorder, the nurse should observe for which sign?
    A. Kernig sign
    B. Turner sign
    C. Cushing sign
    D. Trousseau sign

13. What diagnostic test should the nurse anticipate for pancreas function?
    A. Cortisol
    B. Growth hormone
    C. Fasting blood glucose
    D. Ketones

14. Which of the following are the chemical messengers of the body?
    A. Hormones
    B. Thyroids
    C. Medullas
    D. Pituitaries

15. The creation of new glucose is called:
    A. glycogenolysis.
    B. gluconeogenesis.
    C. hyperglycemia.
    D. hypoglycemia.

# CHAPTER 35 ▶ *Caring for Patients With Endocrine Disorders*

## KEY TERMS

Match each term with its appropriate definition.

1. Cushing syndrome
2. Addisonian crisis
3. Myxedema coma
4. Thyroid crisis
5. Diabetes insipidus
6. Pheochromocytoma
7. Addison disease
8. Goiter
9. Tetany
10. Hirsutism

A. Disease in which an autoimmune response destroys the patient's own adrenal cortex

B. Life-threatening form of hypothyroidism; may be brought on by failure to take thyroid replacement medications

C. Life-threatening response to acute adrenal insufficiency

D. Chronic disorder; the adrenal cortex produces excessive cortisol

E. Benign tumor of the adrenal medulla

F. Enlarged thyroid due to its attempt to produce more TH

G. Extreme state of hyperthyroidism; rare today

H. Insufficient amounts ADH

I. Excessive facial hair

J. Occurs with reduced calcium in the blood

## LEARNING OUTCOMES

1. Describe diabetes insipidus.
2. Describe a thyroid storm.
3. Describe a goiter.
4. Identify manifestations associated with myxedema coma.
5. List steps necessary in the care of a patient having a subtotal thyroidectomy.
6. Describe Cushing syndrome.
7. Identify symptoms associated with Addison disease.
8. Identify nursing diagnoses regarding endocrine disorders.
9. List assessment findings associated with pheochromocytoma.
10. Identify medications used for Addison disease.

# APPLY WHAT YOU LEARNED

You are caring for a patient who presented to the emergency department with extreme fatigue, weight gain of more than 10 pounds in the last month, decreased appetite, slurred speech, and a puffy face. The patient tells you that she is always cold and cannot seem to warm up.

1. What diagnostic tests would the nurse expect to see ordered by the physician?
2. According to the symptoms listed here, is this a case of hyper- or hypothyroidism?
3. What medications and other treatments would the nurse expect to see?

# MULTIPLE CHOICE

Circle the answer that best completes the following statements.

1. A patient, diagnosed with acromegaly, tells you that he is having increased difficulty walking up the stairs at his house. Based on this statement, the nurse prepares a care plan for a nursing diagnosis of:
   A. Disturbed Body Image related to physical changes.
   B. Activity Intolerance related to joint pain.
   C. Pain related to increased weight on joints.
   D. Risk for Injury.

2. Mrs. Kay presents with a temperature of 101°F, malaise, and decreased lung sounds. She has a prescription for L-thyroxine but tells you that she cannot afford the medication. During the assessment, she rapidly progresses to confusion and subsequently becomes unresponsive. You suspect that Mrs. Kay will be diagnosed with:
   A. thyroiditis.
   B. severe bronchitis.
   C. myxedema coma.
   D. sepsis.

3. A patient with a blood pressure of 210/160, severe headaches, diaphoresis, tachycardia, and flushed skin is most likely suffering from:
   A. thyroid crisis.
   B. pheochromocytoma.
   C. goiter.
   D. Cushing syndrome.

4. The nursing intervention that has the highest priority for the patient who has undergone a subtotal thyroidectomy should be:
   A. assess for hemorrhage.
   B. assess for absent bowel sounds.
   C. assess for calcium deficiency.
   D. assess for laryngeal nerve damage.

5. An older woman with hyperparathyroidism is also likely to have:

   A. hypophosphatemia.

   B. hyponatremia.

   C. hypercalcemia.

   D. osteomyelitis.

6. The first priority for treating hypoparathyroidism is to administer:

   A. 500 mL of normal saline.

   B. calcium gluconate.

   C. vitamin D.

   D. calciferol.

7. Treatment for the patient with hypothyroidism is:

   A. 500 mL of normal saline.

   B. lifelong.

   C. vitamin D.

   D. short term.

8. Mr. Tracy was diagnosed with hyperthyroidism 15 years ago. Recently he has been experiencing difficulty breathing and swallowing. You suspect:

   A. thyroid cancer.

   B. hyperparathyroidism.

   C. hypocalcemia.

   D. stroke.

9. Mrs. Kim has been complaining of lower back pain for 6 months. Today her labs show elevated levels of serum calcium, PTH, and alkaline phosphatase. These manifestations confirm a diagnosis of:

   A. stroke.

   B. hypocalcemia.

   C. hyperparathyroidism.

   D. thyroid cancer.

10. Nursing care of the patient with hypoparathyroidism must consider the patient's risk for injury due to:

    A. falls.

    B. tetany.

    C. altered thought processes.

    D. impaired memory.

11. Hirsutism is also recognized as:

    A. excessive facial hair.

    B. loss of facial hair.

    C. balding.

    D. thyroid skin.

12. Cushing syndrome is more common in women between the ages of:
    A. 15 and 30.
    B. 30 and 50.
    C. 25 and 40.
    D. 30 and 45.

13. Hypercalcemia may lead to kidney stones, which are also known as:
    A. calculi.
    B. boils.
    C. striations.
    D. cysts.

14. Nursing care for a patient with hypothermia would include:
    A. applying cool compresses.
    B. using a window fan to circulate the air.
    C. avoiding drafts.
    D. removing blankets.

15. The term *euthyroid* is used to describe:
    A. balanced thyroid.
    B. hyperthyroidism.
    C. hypothyroidism.
    D. Graves disease.

# CHAPTER 36 ▸ Caring for Patients With Diabetes Mellitus

## KEY TERMS

Match each term with its appropriate definition.

1. Hyperglycemia
2. Diabetic ketoacidosis
3. Polydipsia
4. Gangrene
5. Microalbuminuria
6. Ketosis
7. Polyphagia
8. Diabetes mellitus
9. Somogyi effect
10. Polyuria

A. Group of metabolic disorders characterized by hyperglycemia

B. Life-threatening illness in type 1 DM; characterized by hyperglycemia, dehydration, and coma

C. Morning rise of blood glucose after low levels at night

D. Increased urine output

E. Increased thirst

F. High levels of circulating blood sugar

G. Toxic accumulation of ketone bodies

H. Small amounts of albumin in the urine; the first indication of nephropathy

I. Necrosis of tissue followed by infection

J. Person eats more food due to hunger stimulated by decreased energy

## LEARNING OUTCOMES

1. Identify the key differences between type 1 and type 2 diabetes mellitus.
2. Describe the manifestations involved with type 1 diabetes mellitus.
3. Define *glycosuria*.
4. Identify the four main types of insulin.
5. Describe the onset, peak, and duration of long-acting insulin.
6. Describe nursing implications for administering insulin.
7. Discuss nutritional recommendations for adults with diabetes mellitus.
8. Define *ketonuria*.
9. Identify characteristics of hyperosmolar hyperglycemia.
10. Describe clinical manifestations of peripheral vascular disease.

## APPLY WHAT YOU LEARNED

A newly admitted patient to your unit has had diabetes for 12 years. He is 64 years old and works third shift. He tells you that they order out a lot at work, which usually consists of hamburgers, Chinese food, and pizza. You check his blood glucose, and the meter reads 312 mg/dL. Upon inspection of his skin, you notice that his feet have small sores developing bilaterally. The physician is notified of these results and will be in to evaluate.

1. What dietary teaching could the nurse provide to this patient?
2. What would the nurse expect regarding the treatment of a glucose level of 312 mg/dL?
3. What hygiene teaching could the nurse provide in relation to the sores on the patient's feet?

## MULTIPLE CHOICE

Circle the answer that best completes the following statements.

1. The nurse understands that the patient with diabetes mellitus must be cautious when exercising because:
   A. blood sugar levels may drop rapidly.
   B. hyperglycemia may develop.
   C. insulin dosages need to be increased.
   D. exercise produces fatigue and weakness.

2. The nurse is explaining the action of an oral antidiabetic agent. The best statement that reflects the nurse's understanding is:
   A. the medication increases the production of natural insulin.
   B. beta cells are stimulated to release more insulin in response to hyperglycemia.
   C. oral agents provide long-acting release of previously injected pork insulin.
   D. antidiabetic agents slow insulin production by the pancreas.

3. Jacob is being evaluated for possible diabetes mellitus. When collecting the initial data, the nurse should ask:
   A. "Do you eat a lot of sweets?"
   B. "How long have you been overweight?"
   C. "Do you have to urinate frequently?"
   D. "Have you had this type of blood work done before?"

4. The nurse is discussing hypoglycemic reactions with a family. Which of the following statements made by the spouse indicates further teaching is NOT needed?
   A. "I'll make sure that we have some hard candy at home."
   B. "The coffee will make him wake up real fast."
   C. "His son is going to pick up some hamburgers for later."
   D. "We have some wine in the refrigerator if he gets too sleepy."

5. A newly diagnosed patient with diabetes mellitus is concerned about his children. He asks if they should be tested for hyperglycemia. The correct nursing response is:

    A. "Probably; diabetes may be hereditary."

    B. "Yes, your children will have the same condition."

    C. "No, the disease is caused by a virus."

    D. "It's better to find out now than later."

6. A major characteristic found in type 1 diabetes mellitus would include which of following?

    A. People with type 1 diabetes mellitus are generally resistant to the development of ketosis.

    B. Type 1 diabetes mellitus usually occurs after the age of 50.

    C. Pancreas produces no insulin.

    D. Type 1 diabetes mellitus is considered an autoimmune destruction of the alpha cells.

7. The nurse is teaching a class on the care of patients with diabetes. She states that early signs of diabetic ketoacidosis are:

    A. cool, clammy skin, and nervousness.

    B. hunger, headache, tremors.

    C. dark, scanty urine, and diarrhea.

    D. thirst, dry mucous membranes, and poor skin turgor.

8. A vial of insulin is labeled U-100. The nurse recognizes this as:

    A. 100 mg/unit.

    B. 100 units/bottle.

    C. 100 units/dose.

    D. 100 units/mL.

9. If the nurse needs to decide how soon before a meal to give an insulin injection, which of the following must be considered?

    A. Onset

    B. Peak

    C. Duration

    D. Limit

10. A patient with diabetes is seated in the waiting area of your clinic. He begins to complain of nausea and hunger. You observe that he is sweating; experiencing a few chills; and has cool, pale skin. You recognize that this patient may be experiencing:

    A. hypotension.

    B. hyperglycemia.

    C. hypoglycemia.

    D. hypocalcemia.

11. Which of the following is the correct procedure for mixing insulins?

    A. Inject air into NPH vial, inject air into regular vial, and withdraw regular insulin first.

    B. Inject air into regular vial, inject air into NPH vial, and withdraw NPH first.

    C. Withdraw regular insulin first, and then withdraw NPH.

    D. Withdraw NPH first, and then withdraw regular insulin.

12. A patient is admitted to the hospital, diagnosed with type 2 diabetes mellitus, and scheduled for discharge the following day. The nurse realizes that the short hospital stay is not sufficient for adequate diabetic teaching; therefore, the patient's education should:

    A. include specific, realistic goals.

    B. reflect a complete care plan that can be implanted by the home health nurse.

    C. be concise, comprehensive, and intense.

    D. involve the patient's family only.

13. Mr. Jackson, diagnosed with type 2 diabetes mellitus, is prescribed an 1,800-calorie diet with daily exercise. The patient's assessment data include: T 98.6°F, P 90, R 20, BP 160/98, height 5'5", weight 185 pounds. A dietary counseling referral was requested. The primary goal of nutritional therapy is:

    A. control of dietary intake to achieve ideal body weight.

    B. elimination of simple sugars.

    C. reduction in dietary calories to maintain normal blood pressure.

    D. daily equal distribution of carbohydrates.

14. A patient has been seen by the diabetes education nurse. You determine that additional teaching is necessary when the patient says:

    A. "I may have an occasional beer if I include it in my meal plan."

    B. "I will need a bedtime snack."

    C. "I can eat as much as I want to as long as I cover it with additional insulin."

    D. "I should eat my meals, even if I am not hungry."

15. A 16-year-old male patient has been self-injecting insulin as part of his diabetic management. After evaluating his technique, the nurse identifies a need for additional teaching because the patient:

    A. chose an administration site in the center of the finger pad.

    B. washed his hands before the procedure.

    C. told the nurse that he does not repeatedly use the same injection site.

    D. disposed the needle in a sharps container.

# CHAPTER 37 ▶ The Nervous System and Assessment

## KEY TERMS

Match each term with its appropriate definition.

1. Neurotransmitter
2. Refraction
3. Neuron
4. Ptosis
5. Myelin sheath
6. Synapse
7. Dysphagia
8. Flaccidity
9. Dermatome
10. Spasticity

A. An area of skin supplied by a single spinal nerve

B. Basic cell of the nervous system

C. Occurs as light enters the eye and is bent to focus on the retina

D. Helps a nerve impulse cross the synapse or stops it from crossing

E. Difficulty swallowing

F. Increased muscle tone

G. A white, fatty substance that protects and insulates axons

H. Decreased muscle tone

I. Drooping eyelids

J. A junction between neurons

## LEARNING OUTCOMES

1. Discuss the function of the myelin sheath.
2. Identify the three layers of meninges.
3. Describe the cerebellum.
4. Define *reflex*.
5. Discuss the autonomic nervous system.
6. Identify the primary function of the eye.
7. Identify age-related changes in vision.
8. Identify the primary functions of the ear.
9. Name the cranial nerve X and describe its functions.
10. Discuss aspects of the patient's health history that will be assessed related to the nervous system.

## APPLY WHAT YOU LEARNED

The student nurse is studying the topic of the nervous system this semester. He understands that there are different portions of the brain that have their own action and responsibility to the body. He also understands that there are 12 cranial nerves that play a role in the nervous system and control certain functions as well.

1. What cranial nerves are involved with difficulty swallowing?
2. What cranial nerves are related to eyeball movement?

## MULTIPLE CHOICE

Circle the answer that best completes the following statements.

1. A number of changes in the eye and vision occur with aging. The lens becomes less elastic, affecting near vision. This is known as:

   **A.** myopia.

   **B.** nystagmus.

   **C.** irreversible hyperopia.

   **D.** presbyopia.

2. Normal cerebrospinal fluid has a(n):

   **A.** few WBCs.

   **B.** few RBCs.

   **C.** opaque appearance.

   **D.** dark color.

3. Jeff, who has a head injury, has recovered completely except for trouble speaking. What area of his brain was likely affected?

   **A.** Temporal lobe

   **B.** Broca area

   **C.** Parietal lobe

   **D.** Wernicke area

4. Mrs. Mave, age 65, had a stroke. She is having difficulty understanding what you say or write to her. You suspect what area of her brain was affected?

   **A.** Broca area

   **B.** Parietal lobe

   **C.** Wernicke area

   **D.** Temporal lobe

5. A patient with problems swallowing most likely has involvement of what cranial nerves?

   **A.** VII and XII

   **B.** IX and X

   **C.** I, II, and IV

   **D.** VI and XI

6. Loss of fat and subcutaneous tissue around the eyes generally leads to:

   **A.** difficulty focusing.

   **B.** reduced light entering the eye.

   **C.** decreased peripheral vision.

   **D.** increased risk of infection.

7. Ivan's parents complain of him "zoning out" for periods of time during the day. Ivan has no recollection of these times and sleeps heavily afterward. You suspect Ivan may have seizures. What test would determine if that diagnosis is correct?

   **A.** CT

   **B.** Myelography

   **C.** EMG

   **D.** MRI

8. Which test is used to detect brain cancer, Alzheimer disease, epilepsy, and Parkinson disease?

   **A.** EEG

   **B.** PET

   **C.** EMG

   **D.** CT

9. Tracy, an 18-year-old with epilepsy, is visibly upset when you enter her room. She is crying and states, "I can't get this gunk out of my hair!" You realize that she has just had a(n):

   **A.** MRI.

   **B.** EEG.

   **C.** PET.

   **D.** CT.

10. Mark has been complaining about his eye hurting ever since the motor vehicle crash 2 days ago that broke his windshield. You suspect he may have glass in his eye. What type of test would confirm your suspicions?

    **A.** Visual field test

    **B.** CT

    **C.** Fluorescein stain

    **D.** MRI

11. A neuron is composed of all of the following EXCEPT:

    **A.** dendrites.

    **B.** cell bodies.

    **C.** axons.

    **D.** nephrons.

12. The brain receives about how many mL of blood each minute?

    **A.** 750

    **B.** 500

    **C.** 1,500

    **D.** 250

13. The nurse knows that there are how many pairs of cervical nerves?

    A. 8

    B. 12

    C. 5

    D. 10

14. What is the term used to describe eyelid drooping?

    A. Nystagmus

    B. Ptosis

    C. Dysphagia

    D. Presbyopia

15. In assessing for hearing difficulty, the nurse will ask about tinnitus, which is:

    A. need for increased volume.

    B. ringing in the ears.

    C. need for decreased volume.

    D. wax buildup in the ear.

# CHAPTER 38 ▶ Caring for Patients With Intracranial Disorders

## KEY TERMS

Match each term with its appropriate definition.

1. Concussion
2. Otorrhea
3. Hematoma
4. Intracranial pressure
5. Hemiplegia
6. Cerebrovascular accident
7. Transient ischemic attack
8. Aneurysm
9. Seizure
10. Status epilepticus

A. A brief episode of reversible neurologic deficits

B. Pressure exerted within the cranium by the brain, blood, and CSF

C. A brain attack

D. A brief disruption of brain function caused by abnormal electrical activity in the nerve cells of the brain

E. Accumulation of blood

F. A life-threatening medical emergency that can cause permanent brain damage

G. An abnormal dilation of a cerebral artery

H. Paralysis of the left or right half of the body

I. Brain injury resulting from violent shaking or impact

J. CSF leaks from the ears

## LEARNING OUTCOMES

1. List several nursing diagnoses related to head injury.
2. Identify manifestations of a concussion.
3. Identify the three ways hematomas are classified.
4. Describe altered level of consciousness.
5. Define *brain tumors.*
6. Identify manifestations related to brain tumors.
7. Discuss manifestations of a cerebrovascular accident.
8. Describe a seizure.
9. Discuss collaborative care related to status epilepticus.
10. Describe meningitis.

# APPLY WHAT YOU LEARNED

You are working the triage department in the emergency department when a patient comes to you and tells you that he cannot feel his left arm or leg and has double vision, slight facial droop, and trouble finding the "right" words. The patient has no known allergies that he is aware of and denies chest pain.

1. Based upon these manifestations, what could be the diagnosis?
2. What diagnostic tests would the nurse expect to be ordered?
3. What is the treatment plan that the nurse will implement in this situation?

# MULTIPLE CHOICE

Circle the answer that best completes the following statements.

1. Why is death a concern when discussing a patient who has developed cerebral edema?
   A. There is decreased fluid to the brain, which causes dehydration.
   B. The force of the excess fluid may cause the brain to herniate.
   C. It is irreversible.
   D. If the edema lasts longer than 24 hours, death is inevitable.

2. You obtain the following results of a patient's neurologic assessment: eyes open on command, uses inappropriate words, moves to localized pain. Based on the Glasgow Coma scale, this patient should be placed at:
   A. 9.
   B. 11.
   C. 15.
   D. 18.

3. Andrew Smythe has been diagnosed with a CVA due to an embolism. He has global aphasia and requires moderate assistance with ADL. Which of the following would NOT be an appropriate nursing diagnosis for Mr. Smythe?
   A. Ineffective Tissue Perfusion
   B. Self-Care Deficit
   C. Communication: Verbal, Impaired
   D. Urinary Incontinence, Total

4. Tejas has developed increased intracranial pressure due to an infection. You know to monitor for signs and symptoms of cerebral anoxia because:
   A. infections cause a decrease in blood flow to the brain.
   B. increased ICP creates an increased blood flow to the damaged area.
   C. increased ICP may prevent adequate blood flow to the brain.
   D. cerebral anoxia is a symptom of decreased ICP.

5. Jenny is a 2-year-old child diagnosed with a brain tumor. Which of the following questions would be appropriate to ask the child's mother?

   A. "Has Jenny been having trouble staying awake?"

   B. "Does Jenny have any problems with nausea?"

   C. "Have you noticed any changes in Jenny's speech?"

   D. All of the above questions would be appropriate.

6. Malcolm suffered a head injury after a motorcycle crash. The doctor explains that after a head injury, it is not uncommon for a patient to have one or two seizures. If the seizures occur in a chronic pattern, then the patient will likely be diagnosed as having:

   A. adult-onset seizure disorder.

   B. convulsion disorder.

   C. epilepsy.

   D. seizures.

7. Malcolm has been given a new order for phenytoin 100 mg P.O. b.i.d. You are providing teaching about this medication. What information would you NOT include?

   A. Driving a vehicle is permitted following administration of the first dose.

   B. CNS or vision changes must be reported to the physician immediately.

   C. Good dental hygiene is essential.

   D. Blood levels should be checked on a routine basis.

8. Stephanie is a 33-year-old female who developed meningitis after a sinus infection. She has not responded well to the antibiotics and steroids. She asks if she will return to normal after the infection has cleared up. Your best response would be:

   A. "You should recover without complications."

   B. "There is a risk for long-term problems, such as vision or hearing changes."

   C. "Let me call the doctor so he can explain your prognosis to you."

   D. "You will likely be blind and deaf if you recover."

9. Mrs. Deib is 12 hours status postcraniotomy. Which of the following should be included on her nursing care plan?

   A. Keep the head of the bed at 90 degrees.

   B. Encourage Mrs. Deib to eat her prunes every morning.

   C. Obtain vital signs every 8 hours.

   D. Avoid sneezing and straining during bowel movements.

10. Heather is suspected of having a brain tumor. She has become impulsive and has difficulty making decisions. You suspect that her tumor is located in the:

    A. temporal lobe.

    B. frontal lobe.

    C. occipital lobe.

    D. parietal lobe.

11. During the assessment of a patient experiencing headaches, the patient tells the nurse that she has had headaches off and on during the past several years. She also says that she becomes severely nauseated when the pain of the headache begins. Her only management for these headaches has been sleep. The nurse suspects she has:

A. migraine headaches.

B. tension headaches.

C. cluster headaches.

D. general headaches.

12. The first priority when a patient begins to have a grand mal seizure should be to:

A. time the length of the seizure.

B. administer Valium to stop the seizure.

C. place a tongue depressor in the mouth.

D. maintain an open airway without restricting the patient's movements.

13. Altered level of consciousness is likely to be observed in a patient with:

A. increased ICP.

B. strokes, head injury, or meningitis.

C. any injury that causes a decrease of oxygen or glucose to the brain.

D. injuries that primarily affect the cranial nerves.

14. Which of the following interventions would be appropriate for any intracranial disorder?

A. Bowel management, diuretics, anticoagulants

B. Fall prevention, ADL assistance, bowel management

C. Anticoagulants, fall prevention, ADL assistance

D. Reorientation, caregiver training, fall prevention

15. The nurse understands that which of the following is NOT a likely effect of a traumatic brain injury?

A. Brief change in consciousness

B. Long-term coma

C. Increased athletic ability

D. Death

# CHAPTER 39

# Caring for Patients With Degenerative Neurologic and Spinal Cord Disorders

## KEY TERMS

Match each term with its appropriate definition.

1. Rhizotomy
2. Dopamine
3. Bradykinesia
4. Trigeminal neuralgia
5. Paraplegia
6. Thymectomy
7. Fasciculations
8. Demyelination
9. Sciatica
10. Amyotrophic lateral sclerosis

A. Involuntary contraction of skeletal muscles

B. Destruction or loss of myelin sheath

C. Paralysis of the lower part of the body

D. Surgical severing of a nerve root

E. Slowed speech or movement

F. Pain that follows the sciatic nerve

G. Surgical removal of the thymus gland

H. Characterized by muscle weakness; fasciculations; and muscle wasting of the arms, legs, and trunk

I. Characterized by periodic, severe, one-sided facial pain lasting a few seconds to a few minutes

J. Neurotransmitter that inhibits voluntary motor function

## LEARNING OUTCOMES

1. Define *myasthenia gravis.*
2. Describe Bell palsy.
3. Describe the purpose of plasmapheresis.
4. Identify manifestations related to Parkinson disease.
5. Define *Huntington disease.*
6. Describe ALS.
7. Define *rabies.*
8. Discuss spinal cord injuries.
9. Define *autonomic dysreflexia.*
10. Describe spinal cord tumors.

## APPLY WHAT YOU LEARNED

The student nurse is learning about neurologic disorders. Nursing diagnoses related to multiple sclerosis focus on coping, deficits in self-care, and continuing care. The student nurse is trying to understand this disorder so that he can educate a patient the nurse has seen on clinical rotations.

1. What topics would the student nurse discuss with the patient and family to help them better understand the disorder?

2. What could the student nurse suggest regarding coping issues?

## MULTIPLE CHOICE

Circle the answer that best completes the following statements.

1. Rodney is recovering from a fracture of the $T_3$–$T_5$ vertebra after a fall. He has made significant progress in rehabilitation and is due to be discharged home. The primary nursing diagnosis for his discharge planning will be:

    **A.** Risk for Autonomic Dysreflexia.

    **B.** Risk for Impaired Skin Integrity.

    **C.** Ineffective Individual Coping.

    **D.** Self-Care Deficit: Toileting.

2. The primary nursing intervention for a patient with a newly placed Halo vest is:

    **A.** cleansing the pin sites every 4 hours.

    **B.** inspecting the pins and traction bars for tightness.

    **C.** turning the patient every 2 hours.

    **D.** providing pain relief as needed.

3. Angus is 24 hours status post laminectomy. Which of the following should be documented on the nursing care plan?

    **A.** Remove collar during the dressing change.

    **B.** Ensure the corset is applied correctly.

    **C.** Logroll every 2 hours.

    **D.** Assess patency of the Foley catheter.

4. You are teaching the patient and family about anticholinesterase drugs. The patient needs further teaching if he states:

    **A.** "If I start sweating and my heart rate is slow, I will call my doctor right away."

    **B.** "If I forget to take my dose in the morning, I'll just take it with lunch."

    **C.** "I will be sure to always wear my MedicAlert bracelet."

    **D.** "If I am having trouble breathing, I'll let somebody know right away so that I can get immediate help."

5. A patient diagnosed with multiple sclerosis is being prepared for discharge. The nurse is assessing the patient's home care. The most important question to ask the patient is:

   A. "Do you understand the disease process for MS?"

   B. "Will you be able to prepare a well-balanced meal?"

   C. "Do you have enough financial resources to help you through this crisis?"

   D. "Is there anyone at home who has a cold?"

6. A 32-year-old woman presents to the emergency department and is diagnosed by the physician with a cholinergic crisis. Which of the following represents the most appropriate question in order to gain information about this condition?

   A. "Do you feel short of breath?"

   B. "How much of the neostigmine did you take this week?"

   C. "Have you had any nausea or vomiting?"

   D. "Have you experienced any fast heartbeats?"

7. A mother asks the nurse if her child really needs to receive a tetanus vaccine or if there is some other preventive measure that would be more effective. The best response should be:

   A. "He needs the vaccine."

   B. "The vaccine will decrease his chances of developing tetanus."

   C. "If you clean all of his cuts right away, there really is no need for the injection."

   D. "You won't have to worry anymore about tetanus if he gets the shot."

8. Mr. Jones has been taking Haldol for the treatment of a mild psychosis. He displays a shuffling gait, mild hand tremors, and slurred speech. The nurse knows that these symptoms may be clinical manifestations of:

   A. Parkinson disease.

   B. parkinsonism.

   C. Tourette syndrome.

   D. Creutzfeldt–Jakob disease.

9. The primary nursing intervention during the assessment of a person with a spinal cord injury is to:

   A. ensure that the person's head remains immobile.

   B. assess respiratory status.

   C. maintain the airway.

   D. assess for autonomic dysreflexia.

10. Douglas was in a motor vehicle crash several weeks ago and has now been admitted to the rehabilitation facility for further evaluation of his $T_3$ injury. During his teaching session, the nurse should remind Douglas to:

   A. call the nurse for any severe headache.

   B. report a rise in his blood pressure.

   C. practice using his sip-n-puff–controlled electric wheelchair.

   D. ask for help when ambulating to the bathroom.

11. Wanda had a laminectomy 2 hours ago and is complaining of a headache. You logroll her to inspect the dressing on her back. There is a large amount of clear drainage noted on the gauze. Your next action should be to:

A. remove the dressing to check the incision site.

B. raise the head of the bed to relieve the headache.

C. test the drainage with a glucose reagent strip.

D. call the doctor.

12. A patient with chronic back pain confides to the nurse that his pain medications do not seem to be working, and he is afraid he has become addicted. What is the nurse's best response?

A. "You should go to rehab to get over this addiction."

B. "Tell me more about your pain and how you've been taking the medications. Sometimes people with chronic pain develop tolerance to the medications, not addiction."

C. "You're probably right. You should discuss this with your doctor at your next visit."

D. "We'll get you more pain medication so that you will feel better."

13. The most effective drug for the treatment of Parkinson disease is:

A. Sinemet.

B. Parlodel.

C. Permax.

D. levodopa.

14. A patient with severe muscle spasms from a spinal cord injury calls the nurse for any medication that will decrease the pain. The nurse checks the physician's orders and administers:

A. diazepam.

B. Tensilon.

C. Artane.

D. Cogentin.

15. Julian has a complete spinal cord injury at the level of T1. He develops spinal shock. Which of the following is a manifestation of this condition?

A. Tachycardia

B. Hypertension

C. Diaphoresis

D. Flaccid paralysis

# CHAPTER 40 ▶ Caring for Patients With Eye and Ear Disorders

## KEY TERMS

Match each term with its appropriate definition.

1. External otitis
2. Otitis media
3. Retinal detachment
4. Glaucoma
5. Conjunctivitis
6. Diplopia
7. Cataract
8. Vertigo
9. Age-related macular degeneration
10. Presbycusis

A. Separation of the retina from the choroid
B. Double vision
C. Characterized by increased intraocular pressure and gradual loss of vision
D. Inflammation of the ear canal; swimmer's ear
E. Inflammation of the conjunctiva
F. Common cause of impaired vision and blindness in adults over age 65
G. Inflammation or infection of the middle ear; usually affects infants and young children
H. Clouding of the lens of the eye that impairs vision
I. Type of sensorineural hearing loss
J. Sensation of whirling or movement when there is none

## LEARNING OUTCOMES

1. List several manifestations of conjunctivitis.
2. Describe cataracts.
3. Identify manifestations related to glaucoma.
4. Discuss the assessment of visual fields by confrontation.
5. Discuss the pathophysiology of retinal detachment.
6. Describe macular degeneration.
7. Identify tips to prevent external otitis.
8. Define *tinnitus*.
9. Describe vertigo.
10. Identify nursing diagnoses related to hearing loss.

# APPLY WHAT YOU LEARNED

A 55-year-old male presents to your clinic for a follow-up regarding his blindness. He had a chemical exposure accident 1 month ago and has been trying to adapt to his new lifestyle. His wife and teenage son are very supportive and have modified the house to better assist with his independence.

1. How can the nurse help foster independence with this patient?
2. How can the family ensure adequate nutrition?
3. What services would be appropriate for this patient?

# MULTIPLE CHOICE

Circle the answer that best completes the following statements.

1. The nurse is preparing a discharge instruction sheet for a patient who had ear surgery 2 days ago. Which of the following must be included in this plan?
   A. Take antiemetics t.i.d.
   B. Change the inner dressing daily.
   C. Keep the mouth open when sneezing or coughing.
   D. Do not bathe until released by the doctor.

2. A patient with newly diagnosed glaucoma is receiving eyedrops for the first time. After instilling the drops, you gently hold pressure over the lacrimal sac for 1 minute. He asks you why you are doing this. The best response should be:
   A. "If I pinch the nose, you won't move around as much."
   B. "It will help you see better."
   C. "Pressure over the lacrimal sac prevents the drug from entering your blood."
   D. "I'm sorry. I shouldn't have pinched your nose for such a long time."

3. You are responding to an accident in the hospital kitchen. A coworker is bleeding from her right eye. Upon examination, you see a small shard of metal penetrating her eye through the eyelid. Your next action is to:
   A. irrigate the eye with normal saline.
   B. remove the object, then irrigate the eye.
   C. place sterile gauze over the injured eye and tell her to keep the other eye closed.
   D. take her to the emergency department.

4. A cataract is:
   A. a clouding of the eye lens.
   B. the filling of the space between the lens and cornea with aqueous humor.
   C. an occluded canal of Schlemm.
   D. incurable and leads to blindness.

5. After eye surgery, a patient is instructed not to bend over for a couple of days because:

   A. eye pressure increases when bending at the waist.

   B. the medication will flow out of the eye.

   C. it may cause shooting pains in the eye.

   D. the bending movement will increase the pain.

6. A patient with glaucoma asks when his vision will improve. The nurse responds:

   A. "I don't really know. Maybe you can ask the doctor."

   B. "When the canal of Schlemm opens completely and remains open."

   C. "If you use your eyedrops every day, you should be fine in a month or so."

   D. "Unfortunately, the loss of vision is permanent."

7. Xia Zihuen is a native Chinese woman with a diagnosis of retinal detachment. You are giving preoperative instructions regarding the corrective surgery. You should first:

   A. provide information about the mydriatic eyedrops.

   B. discuss the types of corrective lens available.

   C. explain that perfect vision may not be possible after the procedure.

   D. assess her language skills and educational level.

8. The nurse understands that the patient preparing for ear surgery needs further education when he says:

   A. "I'm disappointed I had to cancel the trip to Spain that was planned for next week."

   B. "I can't wait to take a shower as soon as I get home!"

   C. "I'll be sure to keep the outer earplug clean and dry."

   D. "I will call my doctor right away if I have bleeding or increased drainage."

9. The primary nursing diagnosis for a patient experiencing an acute attack of vertigo is:

   A. Anxiety.

   B. Risk for Aspiration.

   C. Risk for Injury.

   D. Powerlessness.

10. You are teaching a patient the proper positioning of the head for instilling eardrops in his right ear. The correct procedure would be to:

    A. lie on the affected side.

    B. tilt the head backward.

    C. tilt the head toward the unaffected side.

    D. tilt the head forward.

11. Which of the following is least likely to develop sensorineural hearing loss?

    A. Patient with Ménière disease

    B. Patient with a perforated eardrum

    C. Construction worker

    D. Patient on high doses of antibiotics

12. The nurse instructs a patient who is using Betoptic eyedrops to check her pulse 1 hour after instillation of the medication. The rationale for this is:

A. tachycardia is a severe side effect.

B. the medication is a beta-blocker.

C. Betoptic is contraindicated in COPD and heart failure patients.

D. the doctor wants a report on the adverse reactions experienced by the patient.

13. The nurse is conducting a Weber test on a 24-year-old patient. He knows that the test is negative if the patient hears:

A. sound in both ears equally.

B. sound in the right ear only.

C. sound in the left ear only.

D. no sound.

14. Which of the following is most likely to develop external otitis?

A. Olympic swimmer

B. Football player

C. Karate teacher

D. Hairdresser

15. The nurse is demonstrating the assessment of the six cardinal fields of vision in a continuing education class. A student asks, "What is the purpose of this test?" The nurse should state that the purpose is to:

A. determine if the patient has vision in those areas of the eye.

B. determine if the patient is able to follow directions.

C. evaluate eye movement.

D. evaluate healing of the eye following surgery.

# CHAPTER 41  The Musculoskeletal System and Assessment

## KEY TERMS

Match each term with its appropriate definition.

1. Osteocytes
2. Tendons
3. Skeletal muscle
4. Yellow bone marrow
5. Arthroscopy
6. Osteoblasts
7. Red bone marrow
8. Crepitus
9. Ligaments
10. Synovial joints

A. Manufactures blood cells and hemoglobin
B. Grating sound or sensation
C. Uses a flexible fiberoptic endoscope to view joint structures and tissues
D. Found at all limb articulations
E. Connect muscles to bone
F. Cells responsible for bone maintenance
G. Connects bones to bones
H. Cells associated with bone production
I. Contains fat and connective tissue
J. Allows voluntary movement

## LEARNING OUTCOMES

1. Define ligaments.
2. Identify the three types of muscle tissue.
3. Describe abduction and adduction.
4. Describe classification of bones by shape.
5. Identify the purpose of an ESR.
6. Describe calcium testing related to musculoskeletal disorders.
7. Define bone absorptiometry.
8. Describe arthroscopy.
9. Define arthrocentesis.
10. Identify normal phosphorus levels.

## APPLY WHAT YOU LEARNED

A 52-year-old female presents to her physician with complaints of musculoskeletal weakness and difficulty performing some ADLs.

1. How would the nurse assess and grade muscle strength?
2. How would the nurse assess range of motion?

## MULTIPLE CHOICE

Circle the answer that best completes the following statements.

1. The nurse is preparing educational material for older adults at a health fair. Which of the following is a good way to describe the function of bones?
   A. Yellow bone marrow contains fat and connective tissue.
   B. There are four types of bone: long, short, flat, and irregular.
   C. Joints are where two or more bones meet, and there are three primary types.
   D. Bones provide structure and support soft tissues. They also protect vital organs from injury.

2. Which of the following is NOT a type of joint?
   A. Synarthrosis
   B. Bursa
   C. Amphiarthrosis
   D. Diarthrosis

3. A nurse teaches Susan, a 62-year-old patient, about musculoskeletal changes in the older adult. Which of these statements by the patient indicates that further teaching is necessary?
   A. "To protect my bones, I will be careful not to get too much exercise."
   B. "Weight training can help me stay strong and healthy."
   C. "I'm worried about my joint and disk cartilage losing flexibility."
   D. "I know that I am likely to lose bone mass as I age."

4. You are assisting the nurse educator in teaching a class on proper range-of-motion techniques. She asks you to demonstrate the movement of pronation. You should:
   A. move in a circle.
   B. turn your palms down.
   C. bend your ankle upward.
   D. turn your foot outward.

5. Which of the following best describes dorsiflexion?
   A. Movement in a circle
   B. Movement away from the midline of the body
   C. Bending of the ankle to bring top of foot toward shin
   D. Straightening of the ankle to point toes down

6. Why would a physician order an arthroscopy?

   A. To evaluate bone density

   B. To produce computer-generated images used to detect small fractures and bone erosions, to evaluate bone density, and to detect tumors

   C. To use echoes to determine more information about muscle and tendon tears, bleeding into muscle, and joint abnormalities

   D. To identify and repair torn tendons or ligaments, an injured meniscus, inflammatory joint changes, and damaged cartilage

7. The nursing student is helping the nurse prepare a patient for an MRI to help evaluate a soft tissue injury. Which of the following questions is NOT appropriate for the student nurse to ask?

   A. "Are you pregnant?"

   B. "Are you well hydrated today?"

   C. "Are you nervous about this test?"

   D. "Do you have a pacemaker?"

8. The nurse is instructing a patient and his wife about a bone scan procedure scheduled for the afternoon. Which of the following should be discussed during this session?

   A. NPO status should be initiated 8 hours before the procedure.

   B. Patient will have to drink 8 ounces of contrast medium.

   C. The patient should be well hydrated and drink extra water after the isotope is injected.

   D. Radioactive precautions must be taken after the procedure.

9. Maintaining an active lifestyle and performing specific exercises such as weight training are two ways to help counteract aging changes, maintain muscle mass, and prevent:

   A. rheumatoid arthritis.

   B. osteoporosis.

   C. fractures.

   D. myeloma.

10. The patient asks the nurse why she is inspecting and palpating his bones. What is the nurse's best response?

    A. "I am looking for any deformities, tenderness or pain, swelling, and warmth. I'm also checking your range of motion."

    B. "This will help me see if your bones and joints are ok."

    C. "I am checking to see if you will need help with your ADLs once you enter the hospital for your surgery."

    D. "Shhh. I'm trying to hear if you have crepitus."

11. Long bones of the skeleton have two broad ends known as:

    A. diaphysis.

    B. epiphyses.

    C. osteoblasts.

    D. periosteums.

12. The nurse understands that when a joint is bent at the limb, it is:
    A. flexed.
    B. extended.
    C. abducted.
    D. adducted.

13. In understanding muscle strength, a grade of 2 describes:
    A. full ROM against gravity.
    B. passive ROM.
    C. paralysis.
    D. full ROM against full resistance.

14. When a hip flexion contracture is suspected, which test should be performed?
    A. Ballottement test
    B. Kernig sign
    C. Thomas test
    D. Bulge sign

15. When evaluating the toes, flexion means to:
    A. curl your toes.
    B. spread your toes.
    C. remain still.
    D. stand on your toes.

# CHAPTER 42 ▶ Caring for Patients With Musculoskeletal Trauma

## KEY TERMS

Match each term with its appropriate definition.

1. Trauma
2. Contusion
3. Sprain
4. Strain
5. Fracture
6. Compartment syndrome
7. Reduction
8. Hematoma
9. Traction
10. Gangrene

A. Occurs when a bone is subjected to more force than it can absorb

B. Caused by significant bleeding into soft tissue

C. Bleeding into soft tissue resulting from blunt force

D. Tissue death that can lead to amputation

E. Use of a straightening or pulling force to return or maintain fractured bones in normal position

F. Restoration of normal alignment

G. A ligament injury

H. Occurs when excess pressure restricts blood vessels and nerves within a compartment

I. A microscopic tear in the muscle that causes bleeding into the tissues

J. Occurs when tissues are subjected to more force than they can absorb

## LEARNING OUTCOMES

1. Identify characteristics of a sprain.
2. Describe several types of fracture.
3. Describe compartment syndrome.
4. Define carpal tunnel syndrome.
5. Describe phantom pain.
6. Identify ways to decrease fractures in older adults.
7. Describe four types of traction.
8. Identify manifestations of compartment syndrome.
9. Describe a fat emboli.
10. Describe RICE.

## APPLY WHAT YOU LEARNED

A 45-year-old male was admitted for a BKA related to gangrene as a consequence of his diabetes. He lives alone in a two-story home. He is angry as evidenced by his shouting at all staff who try to assist him.

1.  What nursing interventions relate to this situation?
2.  How can the nurse assist this patient with discharge planning?

## MULTIPLE CHOICE

Circle the answer that best completes the following statements.

1.  A patient is admitted to the hospital with a fractured hip. Which of these statements describes the main goal of therapy?

    A.  Alleviating pain
    B.  Maintaining circulation
    C.  Preventing additional trauma
    D.  Increasing mobility

2.  The nurse is discussing discharge instructions with a patient who has undergone a below-the-knee amputation. Which action by the patient would indicate acceptance of the body part loss?

    A.  Verbalizing understanding of the dressing change
    B.  Touching the incision
    C.  Asking questions related to pain medication
    D.  Looking at the amputation site

3.  A cast was applied to your patient's left arm several hours ago. You were asked to teach the patient how to care for the cast. Which of the following statements would indicate that the patient understood your instructions?

    A.  "Could I borrow a hair dryer to speed the drying process?"
    B.  "Wow, my arm is warm."
    C.  "Guess I won't need a sling now that I have this cast."
    D.  "Look at the indentations in this cast!"

4.  The nurse is admitting a patient in the emergency department who sustained an injury while playing soccer. Which of the following clinical manifestations might indicate that the patient's shoulder is dislocated?

    A.  Edema of the upper arm
    B.  Pain radiating to the wrist
    C.  Increased length of the affected arm
    D.  Bruising in the scapula region

5.  Jerry twists his right ankle, injuring several ligaments. This injury is classified as a:

    A.  sprain.
    B.  strain.
    C.  contusion.
    D.  fracture.

6. A patient's wrist is edematous and painful as a result of a sports accident. Initial treatment should include:

   A. elevation and heat application.

   B. elevation and ice application.

   C. elevation and Ace bandage only.

   D. elevation and a splint.

7. A fracture that involves protrusion of the bone through the skin is a(n):

   A. complete fracture.

   B. compound fracture.

   C. greenstick fracture.

   D. oblique fracture.

8. A patient has skeletal traction to her left leg. Appropriate nursing action to assist in transporting the patient to the x-ray department would be:

   A. maintain traction during transport.

   B. remove weights before transporting.

   C. place weights on the bed.

   D. secure the weights on the traction frame.

9. Mrs. Carson has had a right hip arthroplasty. A priority nursing intervention during the postoperative phase is to:

   A. maintain the hip in adduction.

   B. maintain the hip in abduction.

   C. maintain the Buck's traction.

   D. perform active ROM on the right leg.

10. A patient has an above-the-knee amputation resulting from uncontrolled diabetes. The nurse should recognize that the purpose of using an elastic wrap on the stump is to:

    A. prevent pain.

    B. prevent hemorrhage.

    C. prevent edema.

    D. prevent infection.

11. When grading a sprain, Grade II would indicate:

    A. complete tearing of the ligament.

    B. overstretching with mild bleeding and inflammation.

    C. partial tearing with inflammation.

    D. the bony attachment of the ligament is broken away.

12. What type of traction is done by physically pulling on the extremity?

    A. Manual

    B. Skeletal

    C. Skin

    D. Balanced

13. What is a partial separation of the bones of a joint called?

   **A.** Subluxation

   **B.** Internal rotation

   **C.** External rotation

   **D.** Extracapsular

14. Another term for tennis elbow is:

   **A.** carpal tunnel.

   **B.** epicondylitis.

   **C.** arthritis.

   **D.** bursitis.

15. Phantom pain is associated with which surgical procedure?

   **A.** Arthroscopy

   **B.** Biopsy

   **C.** Amputation

   **D.** Replacement

# CHAPTER 43 ▶ Caring for Patients With Musculoskeletal Disorders

## KEY TERMS

Match each term with its appropriate definition.

1. Pathologic fractures
2. Gout
3. Kyphosis
4. Rheumatoid arthritis
5. Arthroplasty
6. Systemic lupus erythematosus
7. Arthritis
8. Osteomyelitis
9. Osteoporosis
10. Arthralgia

A. Loss of bone mass
B. Chronic inflammatory connective tissue disease
C. Literally, inflammation of a joint
D. Joint replacement
E. Fractures that occur with minimal or no trauma
F. Results from an accumulation of uric acid crystals in the joints
G. Increased thoracic curvature
H. Systemic connective tissue inflammatory disorder
I. Infection of the bone
J. Joint pain

## LEARNING OUTCOMES

1. Discuss complications of osteoporosis.
2. Identify the pathophysiology of osteomyelitis.
3. Describe osteoarthritis.
4. Define rheumatoid arthritis.
5. Describe lupus.
6. Define fibromyalgia.
7. Discuss the relationship between race and the risk of osteoporosis.
8. Identify multisystem effects of lupus.
9. Identify manifestations of rheumatoid arthritis.
10. Define arthralgia.

# APPLY WHAT YOU LEARNED

A 44-year-old male has just had his second total knee replacement. He is preparing for discharge and is offering no complaints of pain, only minor discomfort with movement. He is scheduled for physical therapy as an outpatient. He resides on a first-floor apartment with his wife.

1. Identify some teaching that the nurse will be doing with this patient prior to discharge.

2. How can the nurse ensure that the patient and his wife understand the discharge instructions?

# MULTIPLE CHOICE

Circle the answer that best completes the following statements.

1. Mrs. Montez, age 58, is diagnosed with osteoporosis. The teaching plan should include which of the following points?
   A. Increase weight-bearing exercises.
   B. Increase isometric exercises.
   C. Reduce calcium intake.
   D. Increase protein intake.

2. The nurse informs a patient with osteoporosis that a new drug has been prescribed to inhibit bone resorption. Which of the following medications has this action?
   A. Sodium fluoride
   B. Calcium carbonate
   C. Estrogen
   D. Alendronate

3. Hanna is diagnosed with SLE. The nurse would be most alarmed if Hanna developed:
   A. painful joints.
   B. severe headaches.
   C. abnormal breath sounds.
   D. weight loss.

4. Hydroxychloroquine has been prescribed for a patient with systemic lupus. Patient teaching should include which of the following:
   A. Have eye examinations every 6 months.
   B. Avoid the use of NSAIDs.
   C. Measure output every 8 hours.
   D. Document daily weights.

5. A patient is prescribed a low-purine diet. The nurse recognizes the need for further teaching if he chooses which food for lunch?
   A. Chicken
   B. Milk
   C. Liver
   D. Corn

6. Your patient has been given a prescription for allopurinol. He calls the clinic to report that a rash has developed on his chest and arms. Which of the following would be the nurse's best response:

    A. "Don't worry, it will go away in a few days."

    B. "Please stop taking the medication."

    C. "Discontinue the drug and make an appointment with your doctor right away."

    D. "Finish taking the pills and then schedule a follow-up appointment."

7. You are teaching a patient about a high-calcium diet. The patient understands the instructions if he tells you that the best source of calcium would be:

    A. a seafood platter.

    B. broccoli casserole.

    C. tofu.

    D. whole milk.

8. The nurse is developing a care plan for a patient with gout. The diagnosis is acute pain. Which of the following interventions should be included in the plan of care?

    A. Increase outdoor activity.

    B. Wrap foot with an Ace bandage.

    C. Keep the foot warm by covering with a sheet.

    D. Administer analgesics as ordered.

9. Joan went on a vacation in the mountains. One month after her return, she developed malaise, fever, muscle pain, and an unusual skin lesion. You suspect that the doctor will treat Joan for:

    A. Rocky Mountain spotted fever.

    B. Lyme disease.

    C. rabies.

    D. malaria.

10. A patient is diagnosed with the most common malignant bone tumor of the long bones. Based on your knowledge of bone tumors, you suspect that the tumor will be classified as:

    A. multiple myeloma.

    B. Ewing sarcoma.

    C. chondrosarcoma.

    D. osteosarcoma.

11. The nurse is reviewing a patient's medical records and notes that the ESR is elevated and the rheumatoid factor is positive. Using this knowledge, the nurse believes that the doctor will make a diagnosis of:

    A. rheumatoid arthritis.

    B. ankylosing spondylitis.

    C. muscular dystrophy.

    D. Paget disease.

12. A low-dose corticosteroid is prescribed for a patient with rheumatoid arthritis. The primary function of this medication is to:

A. inhibit prostaglandin synthesis.

B. slow or prevent joint destruction.

C. rapidly reduce pain and inflammation.

D. reduce infection.

13. The nurse is educating a patient who has just been diagnosed with Paget disease. The nurse understands that the patient needs more teaching when she says:

A. "I understand that one of my goals is to manage and minimize symptoms."

B. "I understand that I got this disease because I have been smoking cigarettes for the past 10 years."

C. "My skin feels warm because more blood is flowing to the affected area."

D. "I can expect to get shorter because of this disease."

14. A pregnant woman is recommended to have a calcium intake of:

A. 400 mg.

B. 1,000 to 1,300 mg.

C. 800 to 1,200 mg.

D. 1,000 mg.

15. Foods high in calcium include all of the following EXCEPT:

A. milk.

B. broccoli.

C. tofu.

D. oranges.

# CHAPTER 44

# The Integumentary System and Assessment

## KEY TERMS

Match each term with its appropriate definition.

1. Alopecia
2. Epidermis
3. Cyanosis
4. Dermis
5. Erythema
6. Pallor
7. Jaundice
8. Clubbing
9. Lentigines
10. Macule

A. Flat, nonpalpable change in skin color

B. Reddening of the skin

C. Angle of nail base is greater than 180 degrees

D. Outermost part of the skin, made of epithelial cells

E. Paleness of skin

F. Hyperpigmentation; *liver spots*

G. Hair loss

H. Yellow-to-orange color visible in the skin and mucous membranes

I. Deeper layer of skin made up of a flexible connective tissue

J. Bluish discoloration of the skin and mucous membranes

## LEARNING OUTCOMES

1. Identify the function of the epidermis.
2. Identify the function of the dermis.
3. Describe three types of glands related to skin.
4. Describe a vesicle.
5. Discuss keloids.
6. Define clubbing.
7. Describe a biopsy.
8. Identify the purpose of a culture and sensitivity test related to the skin.
9. Describe a patch test.
10. Discuss factors related to the color of the skin.

## APPLY WHAT YOU LEARNED

Kate, a 64-year-old patient, is worried about how her skin is changing as she ages. The nurse is helping her learn more about normal age-related changes.

1. What age-related skin changes should the nurse discuss with Kate?

2. Just as she does with her patients of all ages, what are several types of lesions the nurse should instruct Kate to watch for?

## MULTIPLE CHOICE

Circle the answer that best completes the following statements.

1. Caucasians have a pinkish skin tone because of:
   A. profuse erythema.
   B. blood leakage.
   C. red blood cells underneath skin.
   D. melanin.

2. The nurse is reviewing a patient's record and notes that he is at higher risk for skin cancer. Based on her knowledge of this condition, the nurse does NOT expect to find which of the following risk factors documented in the patient's record?
   A. The patient has blue eyes.
   B. The patient is 60 years of age.
   C. There is a family history of skin cancer.
   D. The patient has a dark skin tone.

3. During inspection of a patient's skin, the nurse observes an irregularly shaped, heavily pigmented *mole*. The nurse's next action should be to:
   A. ask the patient if he is aware of the mole.
   B. document the size, color, and appearance of the mole in the chart.
   C. notify the physician immediately.
   D. check the medical history in the records.

4. The nurse receives report that her new patient has scaly skin. What does she expect to see when she goes to assess the patient?
   A. An elevated, pus-filled vesicle with a circumscribed border
   B. A translucent, dry, paper-like skin surface
   C. Shedding flakes of greasy, keratinized skin tissue
   D. A deep, irregularly shaped area of skin loss extending into the dermis

5. The patient reports a rough, thickened, hardened area of epidermis. She says she has been scratching this area a lot recently. What will the nurse know to identify this type of lesion as?
   A. Keloid
   B. Lichenification
   C. Scar
   D. Atrophy

6. Jared, a student nurse, is preparing a handout for a health fair he and his classmates will be attending. What is the best way Jared can explain the function of hair?

   **A.** It secretes sebum, which lubricates skin and plays a role in killing bacteria.

   **B.** It transmits messages via nerve endings to the central nervous system.

   **C.** Its function is unknown.

   **D.** It cushions the scalp. Eyelashes and cilia protect the body from foreign particles. It provides insulation in cold weather.

7. Randy, age 45, has been diagnosed with cirrhosis of the liver. He has a yellow pigment to his skin. You know this is called:

   **A.** jaundice.

   **B.** melaninic.

   **C.** keratotic.

   **D.** cyanotic.

8. You notice that your patient's oxygen is not connected. His lips are starting to turn blue, and he is lethargic. As you hook his oxygen back up and call the respiratory therapist, you realize his lips are:

   **A.** jaundiced.

   **B.** melaninic.

   **C.** keratinic.

   **D.** cyanotic.

9. You notice your neighbor, age 57, outside in her garden. When you go outside to talk to her, she seems confused; thinking she may be dehydrated, you check her skin for:

   **A.** bruising.

   **B.** rashes.

   **C.** erythema.

   **D.** tenting.

10. Red splinter hemorrhages and pigmented bands on nails are normal in 90% of:

    **A.** Caucasians.

    **B.** African Americans.

    **C.** Hispanics.

    **D.** Chinese.

11. Reddening of the skin is known as:

    **A.** erythema.

    **B.** cyanosis.

    **C.** blanching.

    **D.** necrosis.

12. The nurse knows that a patient suffering from a liver disorder will appear:

    **A.** jaundiced.

    **B.** cyanotic.

    **C.** pallor.

    **D.** necrotic.

13. An insect bite or a hive will leave a mark known as a:
    A. nodule.
    B. pustule.
    C. wheal.
    D. macule.

14. The outermost part of the skin is:
    A. melanin.
    B. epidermis.
    C. dermis.
    D. glands.

15. Which gland secretes sebum?
    A. Apocrine
    B. Eccrine
    C. Sebaceous
    D. Thyroid

# CHAPTER 45

*Caring for Patients With*
*Skin Disorders*

## KEY TERMS

Match each term with its appropriate definition.

1. Pruritus
2. Cellulitis
3. Herpes zoster
4. Acne
5. Basal cell carcinoma
6. Pediculosis
7. Melanoma
8. Herpes simplex
9. Warts
10. Folliculitis

A. Fever blister or cold sore

B. Type of skin cancer that arises from melanocytes

C. Infection at skin surface extending into hair follicle

D. Shingles

E. Type of skin cancer that begins in the basal cell layer of the epidermis

F. Subjective itching sensation

G. Skin disorder of the sebaceous glands

H. Infestation with lice

I. Lesions caused by HPV

J. Diffuse inflammation of the skin layers

## LEARNING OUTCOMES

1. Define psoriasis.
2. Describe contact dermatitis.
3. Discuss cellulitis.
4. Describe folliculitis.
5. Define basal cell carcinoma.
6. Identify methods to prevent skin cancer.
7. Discuss the pathophysiology of pressure ulcers.
8. Identify the four stages of pressure ulcers.
9. Describe melanoma.
10. Define nevi.

## APPLY WHAT YOU LEARNED

A 24-year-old female presents to the clinic with a growth on her nose. She states that she does not sun tan; rather, she opts for the tanning salon. She denies using any sunscreen or other protection while in the tanning bed. She is concerned about her appearance and does not believe the growth could be cancerous.

1. Describe the ABCDE rule according to the American Cancer Society.
2. What type of cancer is this patient manifesting?
3. What preventative measures can the nurse explain to this patient?

## MULTIPLE CHOICE

Circle the answer that best completes the following statements.

1. Mr. Williams is admitted to the hospital for treatment of acute cellulitis caused by a spider bite. He asks the nurse to explain what the term means. The nurse plans to base his response on his understanding that cellulitis is a(n):

   A. skin infection that extends into the subcutaneous tissue.

   B. acute superficial infection.

   C. inflammation of the epidermis.

   D. epidermal infection caused by *Staphylococcus*.

2. The nurse is assessing a patient and notices eczema on the back of his neck and bilateral knees. Based on her knowledge of this condition, the nurse expects to find:

   A. gray areas of plaque.

   B. a diffuse red rash.

   C. discoloration and pitting edema.

   D. silvery-white scaly patches.

3. The physician has just diagnosed a patient with herpes simplex. The nurse expects the medication ordered will be:

   A. triple antibiotic.

   B. Bactroban.

   C. acyclovir.

   D. actinex.

4. Retin-A is prescribed for the treatment of acne. The nurse questions the order if the medication is ordered for a:

   A. 12-year-old female diagnosed with asthma.

   B. 15-year-old male diagnosed with cystic fibrosis.

   C. 20-year-old female diagnosed with eczema.

   D. 25-year-old male diagnosed with HIV.

5. Marvin states he will not go to the prom because of his acute acne. The most appropriate response by the nurse would be:

   A. "Lots of kids your age have zits. That's no reason to stay at home."

   B. "Can't you get a date?"

   C. "I can tell this upsets you. Please tell me more."

   D. "The lesions will be cleared by prom time next year."

6. Ms. Taylor has a fungal infection. Which of the following has the highest priority when teaching the patient about the disease?

   A. Take the medication as ordered.

   B. Take the medication on an empty stomach.

   C. Wash hands before eating a meal.

   D. The disease is incurable.

7. What is one of the most effective methods of reducing the spread of infections of the skin?

   A. Reminding patients that they must take their antibiotics exactly as prescribed

   B. Carefully applying gloves with any patient contact

   C. Avoiding skin-to-skin contact

   D. Carefully and consistently performing hand hygiene

8. Discharge instructions for a patient diagnosed with cellulitis should include:

   A. apply cool compresses t.i.d.

   B. discontinue the medication when the symptoms disappear.

   C. cover draining lesions with a sterile dressing.

   D. keep skin moist at all times.

9. Mr. Yale is diagnosed with basal cell carcinoma of the left cheek. Which of the following statements by the patient indicates a need for further teaching?

   A. "I need to wear a hat when I go outside in the sun."

   B. "I need to get my affairs in order, since I don't have much time left."

   C. "The cancer can return after treatment."

   D. "The treatment is usually effective."

10. A neighbor calls one evening and asks you to look at her child's head. When you ask about the problem, the neighbor says that "rice grains" are stuck to the roots of the hair. From your knowledge of lice, you would anticipate that a physician will diagnose:

    A. scabies.

    B. *Pediculosis corporis*.

    C. *Pediculosis capitis*.

    D. tinea pedis.

11. The nurse knows that another word used to describe dry skin is:

    A. pruritus.

    B. xerosis.

    C. xerostoma.

    D. cyanosis.

12. A common medication used in the treatment of acne is:

    A. Accutane.

    B. aspirin.

    C. Allopurinol.

    D. Arimidex.

13. Shingles is a viral infection also known as:

    A. herpes simplex 1.

    B. herpes simplex 2.

    C. herpes zoster.

    D. herpes simplex 4.

14. Which of the following is a parasite?

    A. Lice

    B. Warts

    C. Staphylococcus

    D. Streptococcus

15. A complementary therapy used to treat boils is:

    A. green root.

    B. licorice root.

    C. tea tree oil.

    D. coffee bean oil.

## KEY TERMS

Match each term with its appropriate definition.

1. Eschar
2. Keloid
3. Hypertrophic scar
4. Full-thickness burn
5. Superficial burn
6. "Rule of nines"
7. Burn shock
8. Contracture
9. Debridement
10. Burn

A. Overgrowth of dermal tissue that remains within the boundaries of the wound

B. Type of hypovolemic shock

C. Removal of dead tissue from wound

D. Scar that extends beyond the boundaries of the original wound

E. Permanent shortening of connective tissue related to a burn wound

F. Hard crust that forms over the burn wound

G. Involves only the epidermal layer

H. Occurs when a transfer of energy from a heat source to the human body results in tissue loss, damage, or irreversible destruction

I. Involves all layers of skin; may extend to subcutaneous fat, muscle, bone

J. Rapid method of estimating the extent of partial- and full-thickness burns

## LEARNING OUTCOMES

1. Discuss causative agents related to burns.
2. Describe the "rule of nines."
3. Describe Curling ulcer.
4. Describe the process of debridement.
5. Identify initial focus assessments regarding major burns.
6. Identify nursing diagnoses regarding burn patients.
7. Discuss the open and closed methods of wound dressing.
8. Identify nursing implications and patient teaching related to silver nitrate.
9. Identify diagnostic testing used to assess and monitor burns.
10. Identify aspects of patient and family teaching related to burn care.

# APPLY WHAT YOU LEARNED

A 42-year-old male presents to the emergency department after being burned by a chemical at work. The burns appear only on the patient's face. He was wearing goggles, hat, gloves, and long sleeves while working with this chemical.

1. Using the "rule of nines," what percentage of his body is burned?
2. What treatment would the nurse expect to see ordered?

# MULTIPLE CHOICE

Circle the answer that best completes the following statements.

1. A patient sustains partial- and full-thickness burns over 45% of his body. The nursing care immediately following this burn injury is:

   A. prevention of infection.

   B. fluid resuscitation.

   C. preservation of body image.

   D. maintenance of urinary output.

2. The nurse describes the patient's burn injury in the medical record as "pale, waxy and moist, with large blister formation." The patient states that the pain is a 5 on a scale from 0 to 10. The depth of injury is most likely:

   A. full thickness.

   B. superficial.

   C. superficial partial thickness.

   D. deep partial thickness.

3. The emergent stage of burn injury treatment includes:

   A. closure of the burn wound.

   B. wound debridement.

   C. estimating the extent of the burn.

   D. skin grafting.

4. Mr. Andrews, age 68, is receiving fluid resuscitation of lactated Ringer's solution at 250 mL/hr. Which of the following indicates a complication of fluid therapy?

   A. Urinary output of 50 mL/hr

   B. Complaints of abdominal pain

   C. Crackles in lung bases

   D. Edema in the burn areas

5. A major complication of a severe burn is infection. If all of the following nursing interventions are placed on the care plan, which would be the highest priority?

   A. Monitor and record body temperature every 2 hours.

   B. Review WBC counts.

   C. Maintain a high-calorie diet.

   D. Use aseptic technique.

6. A 7-year-old child sustains a thermal burn to her face when she trips over an open gas heater. Your first action should be to:

   A. determine the depth of the burn.

   B. assess the respiratory status.

   C. provide pain medication.

   D. read the doctor's orders.

7. Your patient is receiving Ensure at 60 mL/hr via a nasogastric tube. Which of the following interventions should be written on the nursing care plan?

   A. Record daily weights.

   B. Replace feeding tube every 24 hours.

   C. Administer a stool softener once a day.

   D. Increase the rate when the patient complains of hunger.

8. Mrs. Jones has sustained burns over 55% of her body. She complains of nausea and has been throwing up a dark green fluid. Your next action would be to:

   A. assess bowel sounds.

   B. insert a nasogastric tube.

   C. administer an antiemetic.

   D. notify the charge nurse.

9. The nurse is reviewing the lab work for a patient with severe burns over 60% of his body. The HGB is 10.8 and the HCT is 55%. The nurse recognizes that these lab values may indicate:

   A. blood loss.

   B. nutritional deficit.

   C. hemolysis and fluid shifts.

   D. infection.

10. A patient is complaining of severe pain after receiving partial- and full-thickness burns to her chest and lower extremities. The nurse expects to administer medication by the:

    A. intravenous route.

    B. intramuscular route.

    C. subcutaneous route.

    D. oral route.

11. Silver nitrate wet dressings are used as a topical treatment for a patient with a full-thickness burn to the left arm. Patient teaching should include which of the following:

    A. The treatment will be painful.

    B. The dressing will be removed every 2 hours.

    C. The dressing will feel warm.

    D. The treatment will cause the skin to turn black.

12. A primary goal of the rehabilitative stage of burn management should be to:

    A. prevent contractures.

    B. prevent infection.

    C. manage the pain.

    D. increase the nutritional status.

13. You have been assigned to assist the physician in the debridement of a burn wound located on a patient's forehead. Which of the following actions would NOT be appropriate for this patient?

   A. Administer pain medications 30 minutes before the procedure.

   B. Wash the wound with mild soap.

   C. Provide a pair of surgical scissors to remove eschar.

   D. Trim any hair that might interfere with the procedure.

14. Mr. Kaiser will be going to surgery for an autograft. He asks the nurse, "Where does the doctor get the graft material?" The nurse should state:

   A. "We have the local university tissue bank send a piece from a cadaver."

   B. "The surgeon will take a piece of skin from your thigh."

   C. "Your daughter has already volunteered to provide a graft."

   D. "The graft is usually taken from a pig skin."

15. A patient with 60% burn injuries will be receiving a nutritional diet. You expect that the physician will initially order:

   A. a 2,000-calorie, high-protein, high-carbohydrate, low-fat diet.

   B. a low-carbohydrate diet.

   C. enteral feedings through a small-bore tube.

   D. gastrostomy feedings.

# CHAPTER 47 ▶ *Mental Health and Assessment*

## KEY TERMS

Match each term with its appropriate definition.

1. Insight
2. Concrete thinking
3. Neurotransmitter
4. Neuron
5. Synapse
6. Stigma
7. Psychosocial
8. Culture
9. Holistic care
10. Family

A. Chemical messengers that conduct impulses from one neuron to the next

B. Attitudes, beliefs, customs, and behaviors passed from one generation to the next

C. Nerve cell

D. Self-understanding

E. Group of people who live together or in close contact and who take care of each other

F. Thought processes that are literal or without creativity

G. Negative attitude marking people with certain conditions as less valuable

H. Space between the axon and its target cell's dendrite

I. Refers to things that affect psychologic and social functioning

J. Caring for a person as a whole, including body, mind, and spirit

## LEARNING OUTCOMES

1. Identify the seven aspects of a mentally healthy person.
2. Discuss why insight is important.
3. Identify five neurotransmitters.
4. Describe a synapse.
5. Discuss stigma related to mental illness.
6. Describe psychologic functions.
7. Identify four aspects of self-concept.
8. Identify the five most common mental illnesses.
9. Describe how mental illnesses are diagnosed.
10. List several risk factors related to mental illness.

## APPLY WHAT YOU LEARNED

The student nurse is studying mental health. She understands that it is holistic and individualized. The assessment of a patient with a suspected mental illness relies on subjective and objective data to evaluate the situation. A mental status assessment tool is also utilized for evaluation and treatment.

1. Identify parts included in a complete mental status assessment.
2. What nonjudgmental question could the nurse ask to find out why the patient is presenting to the hospital?

## MULTIPLE CHOICE

Circle the answer that best completes the following statements.

1. Nancy is a 22-year-old patient diagnosed with depression. When assessing the patient's past coping behaviors, which of the following should the nurse ask?
   A. "Why are you depressed?"
   B. "When the stress gets really bad, what do you do?"
   C. "So, what happened this time?"
   D. "Don't you realize how blessed you are?"

2. A neurotransmitter thought to be decreased in depression is:
   A. GABA.
   B. norepinephrine.
   C. acetylcholine.
   D. FTGA.

3. Which of the following questions could help the nurse assess a patient's self-concept?
   A. "Can you tell me your name, today's date, and who the president is?"
   B. "What things are the most important to you?"
   C. "How do you like your new car?"
   D. "How often do you brush your teeth?"

4. One way to assess abstract thinking ability is to ask the patient to interpret a proverb. This simple assessment can shed light on the patient's:
   A. thought process.
   B. emotional state.
   C. life experiences.
   D. behavior.

5. Which of the following is NOT a basic factor in mental health?
   A. Control over one's own behavior
   B. Sense of meaning in life
   C. Owning one's own home
   D. Adequate rest and sleep

6. A young woman comes into the clinic with chronic pancreatitis. She smiles when you tell a joke, but her overall affect is sad. Because nurses treat patients holistically, a priority aspect of nursing in this case is to promote:

   A. an understanding of neurotransmitters.

   B. patient advocacy.

   C. an appropriate strength training regimen.

   D. mental health.

7. Mental disorders are diagnosed according to the diagnostic criteria published in:

   A. *Taber's*.

   B. the *DHHS*.

   C. the *DSM-5*.

   D. the *PDR*.

8. Which of the following is NOT one of the most common mental illnesses?

   A. Psychosis

   B. Major depressive disorder

   C. Schizophrenia

   D. Alcohol abuse

9. In their role as patient advocates, nurses should stop using negative labels about people who have mental illnesses and:

   A. educate the public.

   B. have a staff meeting.

   C. preach to the choir.

   D. educate each other.

10. A more specific assessment that is appropriate for a patient with mental disorders is called a:

    A. psychosocial assessment.

    B. complete assessment.

    C. mental status examination.

    D. focused examination.

11. To think without creativity is known as:

    A. concrete thinking.

    B. abstract thinking.

    C. foolish thinking.

    D. insight.

12. Which neurotransmitter is decreased in Alzheimer disease?

    A. Serotonin

    B. GABA

    C. Acetylcholine

    D. Norepinephrine

13. Information about a patient's family and culture is an important part of the psychosocial assessment because:

   **A.** more than 90% of people who kill themselves have a diagnosable mental disorder that the fami[ ] can tell you about.

   **B.** family and culture affect each person's health attitudes and behaviors related to health and illness.

   **C.** both subjective and objective data are important.

   **D.** it can reveal a history of drug abuse.

14. What percentage of the population is affected by schizophrenia?

   **A.** 1%

   **B.** 5%

   **C.** 20%

   **D.** 40%

15. The nurse can best explain the concept of mental disorders to the student nurse she is working with by saying:

   **A.** "Mental disorders are very complicated and difficult to treat."

   **B.** "Mental health is very important. It involves neurotransmitters and aspects such as self-concept and family support."

   **C.** "Mental disorders are illnesses with symptoms related to thinking, feeling, or behaviour."

   **D.** "You will see a lot of patients with mental disorders. You'll definitely learn a lot as you work with us on this floor."

# CHAPTER 48 ▶ Caring for Patients With Neurocognitive Disorders

## KEY TERMS

Match each term with its appropriate definition.

1. Cognition
2. Delirium
3. Respite care
4. Praxis
5. Illusion
6. Sundowning
7. Procedural memory
8. Declarative memory
9. Reality orientation
10. Beta-amyloid plaques

A. Performance of skills
B. Temporary condition that alters the level of consciousness
C. Misinterpretation of environmental stimuli
D. Aspect of remembering that applies to skills or physical activities
E. Reminders of person, place, and time
F. Temporary patient care for the purpose of giving the regular caregiver time off
G. Aspect of remembering that involves facts and standard learning
H. Increased mental confusion in the evening
I. Buildup of fragments produced when enzymes act on amyloid protein
J. Thinking skills

## LEARNING OUTCOMES

1. Identify characteristics of normal memory lapse.
2. Describe manifestations of delirium.
3. Discuss components of the Mini-Mental State Examination.
4. Define agnosia.
5. Identify common causes of dementia.
6. Define Alzheimer disease.
7. Identify risk factors for vascular dementia.
8. Discuss the differences between delirium and dementia.
9. Identify differences in etiology between delirium, dementia, and depression.
10. Identify medications used in dementia.

## APPLY WHAT YOU LEARNED

While working in the neighborhood clinic, a nurse encounters a 68-year-old male who reports problems with misplacing keys and his watch. Upon further conversation, the nurse notices that the patient cannot recall the current day and is having problems selecting words for conversation.

1. What do the above signs and symptoms indicate?
2. What resources could be utilized for this patient?
3. What nursing diagnoses would be appropriate for this patient?

## MULTIPLE CHOICE

Circle the answer that best completes the following statements.

1. The nurse knows that as the brain ages, it loses neurons, becomes smaller and:
   A. gains weight.
   B. loses weight.
   C. gains capacity.
   D. loses common sense.

2. All of the following are normal memory lapses EXCEPT:
   A. momentarily forgetting the date.
   B. losing track of what you planned to say.
   C. forgetting where you left your keys.
   D. forgetting how to use numbers.

3. All of the following are frequent causes of delirium EXCEPT:
   A. gout.
   B. heart disease.
   C. psychosocial stressors.
   D. infections.

4. What is the tool used to assess the mental state of patients?
   A. MSDS
   B. MDS
   C. MMSE
   D. MRSA

5. The nurse understands that a disturbance in understanding or expressing language is:
   A. aphasia.
   B. apraxia.
   C. agnosia.
   D. asystole.

6. The following are types of dementia EXCEPT:

    A. vascular.

    B. Lewy body.

    C. Alzheimer.

    D. congenital.

7. A patient presents to the clinic with a history of smoking, HTN, hyperlipidemia, CAD, and DM. The nurse understands that this patient is at risk for:

    A. vascular dementia.

    B. Lewy body dementia.

    C. Crohn's disease.

    D. Lou Gehrig disease.

8. Which of the following is NOT a characteristic of delirium?

    A. Quick

    B. Slow

    C. Fluctuates

    D. Hyper-vigilant

9. The nurse is speaking with a patient who is having problems with language, memory loss, decreased judgment, and loss of initiative. These are symptoms of:

    A. Huntington disease.

    B. Lewy body dementia.

    C. Lou Gehrig disease.

    D. Alzheimer disease.

10. Another term used for putting everything within reach into one's mouth is:

    A. hypersensitivity.

    B. hyperotitis.

    C. hyperacuity.

    D. hyperorality.

11. The nurse receives report that the patient she is about to take care of confabulates. She understands that her patient:

    A. makes others aware of his problems.

    B. makes policies related to hospital admissions.

    C. makes up stories.

    D. makes contracts.

12. The nurse on the 3–11 shift notices that a 68-year-old female patient has increased confusion after supper. The nurse understands this is characteristic of:

    A. wandering.

    B. sundowning.

    C. sunrising.

    D. depression.

13. The neurotransmitter that is decreased in Alzheimer disease is:
    A. serotonin.
    B. acetylcholine.
    C. pepsin.
    D. leptin.

14. The nurse would expect a patient with dementia to be taking the medication:
    A. Exelon.
    B. Excedrin.
    C. Effexor.
    D. Elavil.

15. The loss of brain tissue will have which of the following appearance on an MRI:
    A. localized folds.
    B. no folds.
    C. superficial folds.
    D. deep folds.

# CHAPTER 49 ▶ Caring for Patients With Psychotic Disorders

## KEY TERMS

Match each term with its appropriate definition.

1. Catatonic behavior
2. Anhedonia
3. Tardive dyskinesia
4. Hallucinations
5. Delusions
6. Dystonia
7. Neologisms
8. Prodromal phase
9. Milieu
10. Affect

A. Sensory perceptions that seem very real but occur without external stimuli

B. Lack of ability to feel pleasure

C. Nonverbal expression of emotion

D. Period of early symptoms

E. Fixed false beliefs

F. Permanent movement disorder with involuntary movements of the face and tongue

G. Marked decrease in response to the environment

H. Therapeutic environment

I. Words that have no meaning to others

J. Muscle rigidity; abnormal muscle contraction

## LEARNING OUTCOMES

1. Define psychosis.
2. Describe a hallucination.
3. Identify the most common thought disorder.
4. Identify several manifestations of schizophrenia.
5. Describe milieu therapy.
6. Identify nursing diagnoses related to psychotic disorders.
7. Identify some outcomes for a patient with schizophrenia.
8. Define neuroleptic malignant syndrome.
9. Describe the prodromal phase.
10. Describe bizarre delusions.

## APPLY WHAT YOU LEARNED

An 18-year-old male presents to your clinic and tells you that he keeps seeing Santa Claus in his living room and everywhere he goes. The patient states that he does not intend to harm himself or anyone else. He just wants Santa Claus to "go away."

1.  What might be the diagnosis for this patient?
2.  How would the nurse interact with this patient?

## MULTIPLE CHOICE

Circle the answer that best completes the following statements.

1.  The negative symptoms of schizophrenia involve a deficit or decrease of normal functions and include:
    A. volition.
    B. increased speech.
    C. anhedonia.
    D. sad affect.

2.  Positive (or psychotic) symptoms seem to be an excess or distortion of normal functions and include:
    A. hallucinations and delusions.
    B. delusions and mania.
    C. mania and hallucinations.
    D. anxiety and delusions.

3.  People with schizophrenia in general die earlier than other people do. The largest contributor to this excess mortality rate is:
    A. heart attack.
    B. suicide.
    C. cancer.
    D. renal failure.

4.  The brain disorder in schizophrenia renders many affected people unable to understand that they are mentally ill. The percentage of people NOT receiving treatment at any given time is:
    A. 90%.
    B. 40%.
    C. 54%.
    D. 11%.

5.  A coexisting problem common in schizophrenia is:
    A. homelessness.
    B. anxiety.
    C. chronic disease.
    D. substance abuse.

6. For psychiatric inpatients, the therapeutic milieu should be:

   **A.** simple, safe, and restrictive.

   **B.** restrictive, with flashing lights, and safe.

   **C.** tolerant, safe, and dependent.

   **D.** pleasant, simple, and safe.

7. Antipsychotic medications are used to treat disorders such as schizophrenia that are characterized by psychosis. These drugs are also called:

   **A.** neurostimulators.

   **B.** mood stabilizers.

   **C.** neuroleptics.

   **D.** anticonvulsants.

8. A young woman approaches you on the street asking for your forgiveness. She believes that you are a demon and screams loudly, "I know who you are! You talk to me all the time." You remember from your nursing class that schizophrenia may result in:

   **A.** craziness.

   **B.** delusions.

   **C.** denial.

   **D.** drinking.

9. Roger, age 28 and diagnosed with schizophrenia, stopped taking his medication. What percentage chance is there that he will have a relapse of psychosis within a year?

   **A.** 80%

   **B.** 95%

   **C.** 0%

   **D.** 18%

10. It is important for patients on antipsychotic therapy to be assessed for abnormal involuntary movement with a scale such as:

    **A.** AIMS.

    **B.** MME.

    **C.** HESI.

    **D.** NCLEX.

11. The patient says to the nurse, "I am Wonder Woman!" The nurse recognizes that the patient has which of the following type of delusion?

    **A.** Grandiose

    **B.** Reference

    **C.** Somatic

    **D.** Bizarre

12. The phase in which the patient experiences early symptoms before a full psychotic episode is:
    A. anhedonia.
    B. prodromal.
    C. preprandial.
    D. postprandial.

13. The nurse understands that signs of EPS include all of the following EXCEPT:
    A. dystonia.
    B. dyskinesia.
    C. akathisia.
    D. dysuria.

14. In understanding the effects of antipsychotics, how long may it take for the medications to achieve their full effect?
    A. 4 weeks or longer
    B. Up to 2 days
    C. 6 months or longer
    D. Up to 1 year

15. The inability to sit still is known as:
    A. akathisia.
    B. dysphagia.
    C. arthralgia.
    D. dystonia.

## KEY TERMS

Match each term with its appropriate definition.

1. Mood
2. Affect
3. Psychomotor retardation
4. MAOIs
5. Kindling process
6. Electroconvulsive therapy
7. Distractibility
8. Pressured speech
9. Hypomania
10. Suicidal ideation

A. Generalized slowing of physical and mental activity associated with mental processes

B. Induces a generalized seizure

C. The emotions a person is currently expressing

D. A pervasive and sustained emotion that influences how a person perceives the world

E. So fast and determined that it is difficult to interrupt

F. Episode of abnormally elevated, expansive, or irritable mood; may last 4 days and has no psychotic symptoms

G. Block the enzyme monoamine oxidase that breaks down neurotransmitters in brain synapses

H. Suicidal thinking

I. Repeated stimulus of brain neurons by stress; may make neurons increasingly likely to fire after smaller and smaller stimuli

J. Evidenced by an inability to screen out excess or irrelevant sensory stimuli

## LEARNING OUTCOMES

1. Identify four types of mood.
2. Identify risk factors for depression.
3. Describe psychomotor agitation.
4. Identify protective factors for suicide.
5. Define suicide.
6. Identify side effects related to anticholinergic drugs.
7. Identify foods to avoid when taking MAOIs.
8. Discuss ECT.
9. Describe manifestations of bipolar disorder.
10. Identify patient teaching related to lithium.

# APPLY WHAT YOU LEARNED

A 62-year-old female has been widowed for about 1 year and recently had a stroke that left her paralyzed on her left side. She is currently residing in a nursing home and has no other family. She does not leave her room and keeps telling staff members she wishes that "God would take me already."

1. How would the nurse talk to this patient who is feeling hopeless?
2. What is the first question the nurse should ask this patient?

# MULTIPLE CHOICE

Circle the answer that best completes the following statements.

1. Diane, age 30, comes into the clinic stating, "I'm so depressed!" The nurse knows that risk factors for depression include all of the following EXCEPT:
   A. female gender.
   B. family history of depression.
   C. substance abuse.
   D. recent pregnancy.

2. Brain imaging technology that shows abnormal function in the prefrontal cortex of the cerebrum and in the limbic system during depressive episodes is called:
   A. PET.
   B. CAT.
   C. EEG.
   D. PCT.

3. A major life stressor precedes the first major depressive episode for many people. The average age of onset is in the:
   A. teenage years.
   B. mid-30s.
   C. mid-20s.
   D. senior years.

4. What percentage of childbearing women experience a major depressive episode during pregnancy or within the 4 weeks following delivery?
   A. 0.01 to 0.05%
   B. 3 to 6%
   C. 12%
   D. 36%

5. The nurse knows that it is important to educate patients, their families, and communities about depression, its outcomes, and treatments. The most important benefit of this knowledge is that it can help people comply with treatment, be free from unnecessary guilt, and maintain:

   A. a healthy lifestyle.

   B. their jobs.

   C. faith.

   D. hope.

6. More Americans die each year from suicide than from homicide. Suicide rates are highest among:

   A. older adults.

   B. children.

   C. teenagers.

   D. middle-aged adults.

7. Most antidepressants act on which two major brain neurotransmitters that regulate mood?

   A. Serotonin and dopamine

   B. GABA and norepinephrine

   C. Serotonin and norepinephrine

   D. Norepinephrine and dopamine

8. Patients tend to have better outcomes when they are treated with a combination of medications and:

   A. group therapy.

   B. psychotherapy.

   C. music therapy.

   D. cognitive therapy.

9. Unwarranted optimism, grandiosity, and poor judgment characterize:

   A. depressive disorder.

   B. paranoid disorder.

   C. sleep disorder.

   D. bipolar disorder.

10. Psychosocial factors are important in the timing of manic episodes, and stressful events may precede them. Mania is a:

    A. physical condition.

    B. medicinal condition.

    C. biologic condition.

    D. mental condition.

11. The nurse understands that if a patient is euthymic, the patient is:

    A. in the normal range.

    B. psychotic.

    C. depressed.

    D. irritated.

12. A patient who is experiencing no pleasure is suffering from:
    A. psychomotor retardation.
    B. anhedonia.
    C. psychomotor agitation.
    D. depression.

13. An average of how many Americans die from suicide each day?
    A. 50
    B. 100
    C. 85
    D. 245

14. The nurse understands that treatment with ECT involves:
    A. several sessions with a psychiatrist.
    B. magnetic impulses applied to the prefrontal cortices.
    C. generalized paralysis.
    D. application of electrical current to the brain.

15. The term *pressured speech* is related to:
    A. stress.
    B. depression.
    C. anger.
    D. mania.

## KEY TERMS

Match each term with its appropriate definition.

1. Anxiety
2. Dysphoria
3. Maladaptive
4. Paradoxical response
5. Derealization
6. Obsessions
7. Compulsions
8. Phobia
9. Coping behaviors
10. Resilience

A. Recurrent and intrusive thoughts that cause marked distress

B. Unhealthy coping behavior

C. A feeling of uneasiness and activation of the autonomic nervous system in response to a vague, nonspecific threat

D. The quality of being hardy or *stress resistant*

E. Contradictory; opposite from expected response

F. A persistent and irrational fear

G. Conscious ways that people deal with stress

H. Repetitive behaviors that a person feels driven to perform

I. Uncomfortable and distressed

J. Experience of unreality, distance, or distortion

## LEARNING OUTCOMES

1. Discuss the pathophysiology of anxiety.
2. Identify factors present with a panic attack.
3. Describe posttraumatic stress disorder.
4. Identify medical conditions associated with anxiety.
5. List several defense mechanisms.
6. Discuss resilience factors.
7. Identify antianxiety agents.
8. Identify several expected outcomes related to a patient with anxiety.
9. Describe OCD.
10. Identify the primary characteristic of social anxiety disorder.

## APPLY WHAT YOU LEARNED

A 32-year-old female presents to the clinic shortly after being honorably discharged from the air force. He has a flat affect and tells you that his mind is "all over the place." He has trouble sleeping and states he is having nightmares.

1. What does the nurse suspect is the diagnosis?

2. What are some treatments appropriate for this patient?

## MULTIPLE CHOICE

Circle the answer that best completes the following statements.

1. A nursing assistant catheterized the wrong patient. The nurse takes her aside to point out her error. This is an example of:

   **A.** adaptive behavior.

   **B.** favoritism.

   **C.** maladaptive behavior.

   **D.** prejudice.

2. George comes to the clinic convinced he is having a heart attack. He says the symptoms started on the way to a very important job interview. You suspect George is:

   **A.** having a case of nerves.

   **B.** looking for attention.

   **C.** having a panic attack.

   **D.** procrastinating.

3. A patient copes with anxiety by deliberately relaxing or practicing deep breathing in situations that he expects will provoke anxiety, thereby interrupting the automatic anxiety responses. This patient is using concepts from:

   **A.** ACT.

   **B.** ADHD.

   **C.** CBT.

   **D.** CHF.

4. CBT, or cognitive-behavior therapy, usually takes about:

   **A.** 1 month.

   **B.** 3 years.

   **C.** 2 weeks.

   **D.** 12 weeks.

5. The nurse knows that all of the following statements by his patient represent irrational beliefs EXCEPT:

   A. "I can't believe I forgot to send in the cupcakes with my son today. Now his teacher will be sure to think I'm a bad parent who can't take care of my child."

   B. "Well, I've never been able to keep a girlfriend, so I'm just resigned to growing old alone."

   C. "With my second son on the way, I know it's going to be a really busy time. I think it would be a good idea to hire someone to clean the house so that I don't have to."

   D. "With my second son on the way, I know it's going to be a really busy time. I will make sure I am up before everyone else so that I have time to start preparing all our meals, and then I will clean while the baby is napping. After the kids are in bed, I can get my studying done."

6. Martha comes into the physician's office visibly upset. All of her VS are increased and she is not able to focus as the physician tries to redirect her. Martha is exhibiting what level of anxiety?

   A. Mild

   B. Severe

   C. Panic

   D. Moderate

7. The limbic structure responsible for coordinating actions of the autonomic nervous system and endocrine system, and which is involved in control of emotions, nurturing behavior, and fear conditioning, is called the:

   A. hypothalamus.

   B. thalamus.

   C. amygdala.

   D. pituitary.

8. Your patient has learned to verbalize his own feelings of anxiety and understand his stress response. This phase of anxiety is called:

   A. family.

   B. community.

   C. stabilization.

   D. acute.

9. Nurses can diagnose and treat the symptom of anxiety:

   A. with MD's orders only.

   B. with health care team's approval.

   C. collaboratively.

   D. independently.

10. Information about the patient's usual coping methods can be helpful in:

    A. administering medicine.

    B. gaining information.

    C. discharge planning.

    D. planning care.

11. The nurse understands that the hippocampus is responsible for:

   A. processing information between parts of the brain.

   B. composing neurons that produce hormones.

   C. coordinating action of ANS.

   D. relaying sensory input from spinal cord.

12. A patient who has a widened perceptual field and increased ability to see relationships among data is in which state of anxiety?

   A. Panic

   B. Severe

   C. Moderate

   D. Mild

13. When someone fears being out in a crowd, they suffer from:

   A. agoraphobia.

   B. apiphobia.

   C. astraphobia.

   D. aviophobia.

14. The nurse realizes her patient needs more teaching about his diagnosis of OCD when he says:

   A. "I can see that my compulsions are unreasonable and excessive."

   B. "I know I perform these behaviors to reduce stress."

   C. "I understand that when my stress levels increase, my coping behaviors will improve."

   D. "My rituals bring me no pleasure."

15. Which of the following is a sedative-hypnotic agent?

   A. Ambien

   B. Inderal

   C. BuSpar

   D. Acetaminophen

# CHAPTER 52

# Caring for Patients With Personality Disorders

## KEY TERMS

Match each term with its appropriate definition.

1. Personality
2. Self-identity
3. Impulsive
4. Inflexible
5. Inappropriate affect
6. Linehan
7. Self-invalidation
8. Active passivity
9. Ideas of reference
10. Parasuicidal behavior

A. Behavior aimed at harming but not killing oneself

B. Cognitive deficit in which patients misinterpret everyday events as having a personal meaning for them

C. The psychosocial traits and characteristics that make a person an individual

D. Part of normal personality development; includes integration of social and occupational roles

E. Leading contemporary theorist on borderline personality disorder

F. Occurs when the patient has an emotional response that is not culturally appropriate for the situation

G. Unable to foresee consequences or control urges

H. Inability to change behavior when circumstances suggest that a change is indicated

I. Failure to recognize own emotions, thoughts, behaviors

J. Failure to work actively on solving own life problems

## LEARNING OUTCOMES

1. List five basic personality traits.
2. Describe the three clusters of personality disorders.
3. Describe several characteristics of a patient with inappropriate affect.
4. Define antisocial personality disorder.
5. Describe narcissistic personality disorder.
6. Describe dependent personality disorder.
7. Identify coping mechanisms for someone who uses self-harming behavior.
8. Define borderline personality.
9. Discuss collaborative care for patients with antisocial personality.
10. List several possible nursing interventions for a patient with disturbed thought processes.

## APPLY WHAT YOU LEARNED

The student nurse is studying personality disorders. The student will be observing patients with personality disorders in clinical next week. The objective for this rotation is to ensure safety within the unit for the patients and staff.

1. How will the student nurse help prevent patients with personality disorders from upsetting the unit?

2. What specific nursing interventions might the student nurse employ to address patients with impaired social interaction?

## MULTIPLE CHOICE

Circle the answer that best completes the following statements.

1. When teaching patient strategies about coping with stress, the nurse uses the mnemonic "A wise mind ACCEPTS." The S stands for:
    A. stimulants are great.
    B. supine position works.
    C. sensations that are intense.
    D. Serax works wonders.

2. Which technique is used to help people who have used self-harm for coping find more enduring and adaptive ways to comfort themselves?
    A. Caffeine
    B. Five senses exercise
    C. Finger paints
    D. Valium

3. A nursing intervention for patients who have thoughts about self-harm or suicide is:
    A. negotiating a no self-harm contract.
    B. administering sedatives.
    C. allowing two visitors every 30 minutes.
    D. maintaining a dimly lit, quiet room.

4. A pervasive pattern of social shyness, feelings of inadequacy, and hypersensitivity to negative evaluation is called:
    A. avoidant personality disorder.
    B. anxiety.
    C. paranoid behavior.
    D. schizotypal personality disorder.

5. Mrs. Jones demonstrates a need to be taken care of, which characterizes:
    A. dependent personality disorder.
    B. anxiety.
    C. affective disorder.
    D. depression.

6. Marsha, age 38, seems overly trusting of her boss. She believes everything her boss tells her and acts on any suggestions she makes. She has alienated all her friends because of her attempts to get attention by whatever means possible. The nurse suspects that Marsha suffers from:

   **A.** narcissistic personality disorder.

   **B.** dependent personality disorder.

   **C.** addiction.

   **D.** histrionic personality disorder.

7. How are personality disorders diagnosed?

   **A.** By looking at level of personality functioning

   **B.** By a PET scan and an MRI

   **C.** By identifying how severely the individual's personality is affected in two dimensions

   **D.** By interviewing the patient as well as friends and family

8. Any judgment about a patient's personality must take into account that person's ethnic, social, and:

   **A.** monetary background.

   **B.** cultural background.

   **C.** emotional background.

   **D.** psychologic background.

9. A patient comes to the clinic crying, "I just left my boyfriend … he beat me every day, I just couldn't take it any more. I'm so weak; maybe if I could take it he would love me more." As a nurse you know the best response would be:

   **A.** "Are you crazy?"

   **B.** "If you go back, he will continue to harm you."

   **C.** "He is an adult and responsible for his own behavior."

   **D.** "Why do you want to go back?"

10. One way a nurse can prevent a patient with personality disorder from disrupting the unit is by:

    **A.** making the unit rules clear.

    **B.** having a conference with staff.

    **C.** A and B.

    **D.** none of the above.

11. A patient who suffers from OCD is in which of the following cluster?

    **A.** Anxious/fearful

    **B.** Odd/eccentric

    **C.** Dramatic/emotional

    **D.** Compulsive/obsessive

12. Someone who laughs when a person dies has:

    **A.** delusions.

    **B.** inappropriate affect.

    **C.** psychomotor agitation.

    **D.** depression.

13. Avoidant personality disorder is characterized by:

   **A.** social isolation.

   **B.** anxiety.

   **C.** powerlessness.

   **D.** fear.

14. The relatively stable way in which a person thinks, feels, and behaves is:

   **A.** personality.

   **B.** egocentric.

   **C.** selfish.

   **D.** normal.

15. When talking with a patient who has a disturbed thought process, always:

   **A.** speak loudly and clearly.

   **B.** laugh and joke.

   **C.** reassure them of their safety.

   **D.** reassure them of their discharge.

# CHAPTER 53 ▶ Caring for Patients With Substance Use Disorders

## KEY TERMS

Match each term with its appropriate definition.

1. Tolerance
2. Abstinence
3. Denial
4. Intoxication
5. Wernicke syndrome
6. Ataxia
7. Withdrawal
8. Impaired nurse
9. Korsakoff syndrome
10. Euphoria

A. Staggering gait
B. Exaggerated feeling of well-being
C. Experienced when use of a substance is discontinued
D. Symptoms caused by vitamin B deficiency
E. Works under the influence of substances
F. Refusal to acknowledge the existence of a situation or feeling
G. Increasing amounts of substance needed to create an effect
H. Complete lack of drug use
I. Group of reversible symptoms produced by use of a substance
J. Alcoholic encephalopathy

## LEARNING OUTCOMES

1. Discuss denial.
2. Identify commonly abused substances.
3. Identify withdrawal symptoms related to alcoholism.
4. Describe characteristics of Korsakoff syndrome.
5. Describe characteristics of Wernicke syndrome.
6. Identify manifestations of fetal alcohol syndrome.
7. Define detoxification.
8. Describe rehabilitation.
9. Describe dual diagnosis.
10. Describe an impaired nurse.

## APPLY WHAT YOU LEARNED

The student nurse is preparing for her community service project. She is required to attend an AA meeting and observe the steps involved. She is feeling a little nervous and does not know what to expect.

1. What stereotypes are created regarding alcoholics?
2. How would the student nurse assess a patient for substance abuse?

## MULTIPLE CHOICE

Circle the answer that best completes the following statements.

1. Drugs that distort the user's perception of reality are called:
   A. stimulants.
   B. amphetamines.
   C. hallucinogens.
   D. nicotine.

2. A medication given during alcohol withdrawal to prevent Wernicke syndrome is:
   A. caffeine.
   B. vitamin B$_1$.
   C. Dilantin.
   D. Valium.

3. A nursing intervention that provides low stimulation for the patient during drug withdrawal includes:
   A. restricting visitors.
   B. administering sedatives.
   C. allowing two visitors every 30 minutes.
   D. maintaining a dimly lit, quiet room.

4. A drug prescribed to deter patients from drinking alcohol is:
   A. Antabuse.
   B. methadone.
   C. ReVia.
   D. Catapres.

5. Mr. Jones demonstrates frequent mood changes with increased alcohol intake. These changes are termed:
   A. labile.
   B. anxiety.
   C. euphoria.
   D. depression.

6. A young male increases his consumption of alcohol from one six-pack to two six-packs of beer per day to achieve the same effects. This action may indicate:

   A. addiction.

   B. intoxication.

   C. tolerance.

   D. dependence.

7. A local maintenance man is frequently seen drinking for hours at the local bar. He refuses to socialize with his neighbors and has been labeled an *angry man*. The nurse is aware that a crucial phase of alcohol addiction includes:

   A. emotional and physical disintegration.

   B. memory blackouts.

   C. loss of control over the decision to drink or not to drink.

   D. a steady increase of alcohol consumption.

8. You remember from your nursing class that the chronic phase of alcohol addiction may result in:

   A. job loss.

   B. suicide.

   C. denial.

   D. drinking in secret.

9. A chronic alcoholic has been admitted to the medical floor for a laceration of the forehead and observation. During your physical assessment, you note the presence of ascites, yellow skin, and severe muscle weakness. You suspect that this patient may be diagnosed with end-stage liver disease known as:

   A. confabulation.

   B. alcoholic hepatitis.

   C. cirrhosis.

   D. portal hypertension.

10. A 21-year-old male was brought to the emergency department by the paramedics. They report the patient was found, unresponsive, lying on a park bench. Their initial assessment noted pinpoint pupils and depressed respirations. The ED nurse suspects that this patient may have overdosed on:

    A. alcohol.

    B. amphetamines.

    C. cocaine.

    D. heroin.

11. A patient is concerned about the withdrawal effects from his use of the drug Ecstasy. He states, "I don't want to start shaking. I've seen it happen with my friend who drank too much." The best response by the nurse would be:

    A. "Don't worry, we'll be right here to watch you."

    B. "You won't have any withdrawal symptoms."

    C. "You should have stopped taking the drug a long time ago."

    D. "You won't have withdrawal symptoms, but you might have flashbacks."

12. At a chemical substance treatment center, the nurse is teaching a family about the importance of understanding drug withdrawal from heroin. He explains that a synthetic opiate will be used to replace the heroin. This drug is known as:

    **A.** methadone.

    **B.** naltrexone.

    **C.** Antabuse.

    **D.** Catapres.

13. You observe that the medication nurse always seems to go to the bathroom after administering narcotics. You also notice that more pain medications are given when that particular nurse is on duty. Your next action should be to:

    **A.** do nothing; it is none of your business.

    **B.** confront the nurse when she comes out of the bathroom.

    **C.** discuss your concerns with your supervisor.

    **D.** continue to watch for more unusual behaviors.

14. The major goal of withdrawal management is:

    **A.** cessation of drug use.

    **B.** protection of society.

    **C.** physiological safety.

    **D.** maintaining sobriety.

15. The nurse establishes a nursing diagnosis of deficient knowledge for a patient during the acute phase of substance abuse treatment. Teaching should include all of the following except:

    **A.** consequences of drug use.

    **B.** reasons behind drug use.

    **C.** coping strategies.

    **D.** recommended amounts of drug use.

# Answer Key

## Chapter 1 Nursing in the 21st Century

### Matching

1. H
2. C
3. J
4. A
5. B

6. D
7. I
8. E
9. F
10. G

### Learning Outcomes

1. Care of adults to promote and maintain health, and, during illness, to alleviate suffering. The focus is on the adult patient's response to actual or potential disruptions in health.
2. To promote and provide care to adult patients, nurses focus on quality and safety via patient-centered care, teamwork and collaboration, evidence-based practice, quality improvement, safety, and informatics.
3. The process of evaluating, monitoring, or regulating the standard of services provided to the consumer.
4. Objectives of an advocate are to communicate with other health care team members, provide teaching to patient and family, support clinical decision making, suggest referrals as appropriate, and identify community resources.
5. Phases of the nursing process are: assessment, diagnosis, planning, implementation, and evaluation.
6. Critical thinking is a process used by nurses to determine a patient's needs and is based on priority. The nurse uses knowledge and experience to develop the appropriate interventions in order to assist the patient to maintain an optimum state of wellness.
7. The nurse has multiple roles, including caregiver, manager of care, collaborator, patient advocate, and teacher.
8. The purpose of HIPAA is to protect each individual's health information while allowing such information to be shared as needed for effective care. By protecting this information, the patient's privacy and dignity are maintained.
9. Ethics is a set of principles of conduct that are concerned with moral duty, values, obligations, and the distinction between right and wrong.
10. Professional boundaries are the limits maintained between a person who is vulnerable and the person who has the power. It is the nurse's responsibility to establish and maintain professional boundaries while retaining an appropriate level of involvement for effective care.

### Apply What You Learned

1. The phases of the nursing process are: assessment, where data is collected; diagnosis, where a conclusion is developed concerning condition; planning, where interventions and outcomes are designed; implementation, carrying out the plan; and evaluation, where goals are analyzed to see if revision or completion has been met.
2. During the evaluation phase, the nurse determines whether the plan was effective. Then it is decided if the same plan is to continue, be revised, or terminated. It is based upon the expected outcomes that were established during the planning phase. Evaluation takes place continuously throughout care.
3. First, only a physician can develop a medical diagnosis. A nurse develops a nursing diagnosis to assist the patient in achieving optimum wellness given the current condition. A medical diagnosis will tell the nurse what the disease is, while a nursing diagnosis will guide the planning of a patient's health care status.

## Multiple Choice

| | | | |
|---|---|---|---|
| 1. | C | 9. | C |
| 2. | D | 10. | A |
| 3. | A | 11. | C |
| 4. | D | 12. | A |
| 5. | B | 13. | D |
| 6. | A | 14. | A |
| 7. | D | 15. | B |
| 8. | A | | |

## Chapter 2  Health, Illness, and Settings of Care

### Matching

| | | | |
|---|---|---|---|
| 1. | J | 6. | C |
| 2. | A | 7. | H |
| 3. | E | 8. | D |
| 4. | B | 9. | F |
| 5. | I | 10. | G |

### Learning Outcomes

1. The health–illness continuum is a representation of health as a dynamic process, with high-level wellness at one extreme of the continuum and death at the opposite extreme. Individuals place themselves at different locations on the continuum at specific points in time.

2. Leading health indicators for *Healthy People 2020* include access to health services; clinical preventive services; environmental quality; injury and violence; maternal, infant, and child health; mental health nutrition, physical activity, and obesity; oral health; reproductive and sexual health; social determinants; substance abuse; and tobacco.

3. Illness is the response a person has to a disease. This response is highly individualized because the person responds not only to his or her own perceptions of the disease but also to the perceptions of others.

4. Some characteristics of a chronic illness include that it is permanent, it leaves a permanent disability, it is caused by nonreversible pathologic alterations, it requires special teaching of the patient for rehabilitation, and it may require a long period of care.

5. Long-term care is for people who are mentally or physically unable to care for themselves independently and may require health care and help with activities of daily living. Patients may remain in these types of facilities for the rest of their lives.

6. Community-based nursing is care that focuses on culturally competent individuals who can help families with their health care needs. It can occur in clinics, day care programs, churches, schools, and correctional facilities.

7. Community-based nursing care settings include county health departments, parish nursing, homeless shelters, crisis intervention centers, ambulatory surgical centers, free clinics, hospice care, and prisons.

8. Patients who would benefit from home health care services are those who cannot live alone because of age, illness, or disability. They may also have a chronic disease or be terminally ill and want to die in their home with comfort and dignity. They do not require inpatient treatment but need assistance such as an outpatient surgical patient might require.

9. Areas to assess for safety in the home include stairs, how people manage their own care if they are alone, smoke detectors, bathroom safety equipment, electrical hazards, fire hazards, infection hazards, throw rugs and clutter, expired medications or those that are inappropriately stored, inappropriate footwear or clothing, inadequate food supply, poorly functioning utilities, signs of abuse or abusive behaviour, and safe handling of medical gases such as oxygen.

10. Suggestions for effective home care include establishing trust, assessing the overall environment, promoting the patient's ability to learn, paying attention to the patient's needs, and being flexible.

## Apply What You Learned

1. The nurse needs to teach the patient about bathroom safety equipment and perhaps have a bedside commode to be utilized on the first floor of the home. The nurse also needs to assess the lighting in the house and open the blinds for better visualization. Ask the patient to repeat instructions to the nurse to verify understanding.
2. The nurse could recommend a senior center so that the patient can make friends and have companionship, a Meals on Wheels program to ensure that the patient is being fed, and home health nursing visits.

## Multiple Choice

| | |
|---|---|
| 1. A | 9. B |
| 2. C | 10. D |
| 3. D | 11. C |
| 4. C | 12. D |
| 5. C | 13. D |
| 6. D | 14. C |
| 7. A | 15. B |
| 8. B | |

## Chapter 3   Cultural and Developmental Considerations for Adults

## Matching

| | |
|---|---|
| 1. C | 6. D |
| 2. J | 7. E |
| 3. A | 8. H |
| 4. B | 9. G |
| 5. I | 10. F |

## Learning Outcomes

1. Culture includes learned behavior, values, beliefs, norms, and practices that are shared by a particular group of people.
2. Health disparities are differences in the incidence and outcomes of diseases and disorders that occur among specific population groups in the United States.
3. Blood transfusions are not allowed, but they will accept autologous blood transfusions. Avoid foods to which blood has been added, such as lunchmeats. Jehovah's Witnesses do not observe national or religious holidays.
4. Health risks for young adults include motor vehicle crashes, use of firearms, substance abuse, sexually transmitted infections, drowning, fire, and occupational accidents.
5. Family carries out the tasks that are necessary for its survival and continuity, such as providing shelter, food, clothing, and health care; sharing money, time, and space; determining the roles and responsibilities of each member; and ensuring socialization of members.
6. The diverse and multicultural nature of the population in the United States requires nurses to provide care that is culturally sensitive while avoiding stereotyping.
7. The young adult is at the peak of physical development. The young adult is at risk for alterations in health from unintentional and intentional injuries, sexually transmitted infections (STIs), substance abuse, and physical or psychosocial stressors. Middle adults may gain weight because they continue to consume the same number of calories while physical activity and basal metabolic rate decrease. Obesity affects all the major organ systems. Middle adults may smoke cigarettes and use a variety of substances.

8. Personal space is important because it allows the patient to establish trust with the health care provider. It provides security, privacy, and a sense of control. Maintaining a comfort zone is important for the patient to be able to communicate more freely and thus improves care outcomes.

9. Social orientation includes a group of beliefs, values, and attitudes about important life events such as birth, death, puberty, childbearing, raising children, illness, and disease.

10. Health risks for middle adults include physical inactivity, obesity, cardiovascular disease, cancer, substance abuse, and psychosocial stressors.

## Apply What You Learned

1. Extended families, skip-generation families, alternative families, and blended families are all represented.

2. These students could be taught the importance of a healthy diet to help prevent obesity, cardiovascular disease, and even certain cancers. They should also be taught about the appropriate amount of sleep to maintain health. Socialization should be taught in order for successful development into adulthood. This age group should also be taught about accident prevention, which will include sports and recreation, and STI prevention.

## Multiple Choice

1. D
2. D
3. A
4. B
5. B
6. C
7. B
8. C
9. B
10. C
11. A
12. B
13. B
14. A
15. C

## Chapter 4    The Older Adult in Health and Illness

## Matching

1. H
2. J
3. F
4. I
5. G
6. B
7. E
8. D
9. A
10. C

## Learning Outcomes

1. Ageism is a form of prejudice in which older adults are stereotyped by characteristics found only in a small number of their age group. Two myths related to older adults are that most older adults live in nursing homes, when in fact only about 5% do, and that most older adults are sick when in fact almost half of all older adults rate their health as good or excellent.

2. Gerontologic nursing is a specialty area in the care of the older adult. Research indicates that the older adult population is increasing more rapidly than any other age group, therefore increasing the demand for this specialty.

3. Cognition is the ability to perceive and understand one's world. It does not normally change with aging. Older adults may take longer to process information and to respond, they rely on lists and calendars more, and processing information is delayed when in a new environment.

4. Erikson would identify the older adult to be in the ego integrity vs. despair and disgust stage. This is where the older adult reflects on his or her life and accepts the past.

5. To encourage reminiscence, the nurse would begin by asking open-ended questions to get the older adult to speak about life events. The nurse could also ask the older adult to look at pictures and tell a story related to that picture.

6. Age-related physical changes in the older adult can include the hair on the scalp thinning, decreased turgor and dryness of the skin, narrowed visual field, decreased sense of smell, decreased cardiac output, decreased gag reflex, and decrease in weight and storage capacity of the liver.

7. Psychosocial changes are life changes affecting relationships, income, or location. Widowhood and retirement are two of the most significant life changes that the older adult must deal with and accept.

8. In teaching the older adult about prevention of accidents, the nurse should remind them to install smoke detectors, not to use throw rugs, to have adequate lighting, and to always wear corrective lenses and hearing aids when driving.

9. Alzheimer disease is the most common degenerative neurologic illness. Symptoms usually seen in the early stages are loss of concentration and forgetfulness. It is not considered a normal part of aging.

10. To improve or maintain an older adult's quality of life, it is important for the person to eat a healthy diet, not use tobacco products, receive immunizations for the flu, and continue with annual screenings to detect chronic illnesses.

## *Apply What You Learned*

1. Instruct the patient and family to keep the house well lit and free of throw rugs. Install smoke detectors and use hand railings in the bathroom/tub areas.

2. When promoting the health of the older adult, it is important to assess mobility for exercising, verify if they have dentures or loose/damaged teeth; review their diet for fiber and fluid intake, discuss neighborhood safety and community events, and evaluate that they have a clean, odor-free environment.

3. Since the patient lives alone, the nurse should ask the social services department to speak with her to make sure that the home is ready and safe for her return. The nurse should also have the dietician speak with her regarding a low-sodium diet related to the hypertension. Another possibility would be for someone from the physical therapy department to give her exercise tips to assist in the reduction of blood pressure.

## *Multiple Choice*

| | |
|---|---|
| 1. C | 9. C |
| 2. A | 10. B |
| 3. B | 11. C |
| 4. B | 12. C |
| 5. C | 13. C |
| 6. A | 14. B |
| 7. A | 15. A |
| 8. D | |

## Chapter 5    Guidelines for Patient Assessment

### *Key Terms*

| | |
|---|---|
| 1. D | 6. A |
| 2. I | 7. C |
| 3. B | 8. G |
| 4. F | 9. H |
| 5. E | 10. J |

## Learning Outcomes

1. The purposes of a patient assessment are to collect subjective and objective data, to collect information about the patient's family and community, to identify past and present behaviors regarding heal care, and to identify data that may suggest risk or actual health problems.
2. Subjective data, or symptoms, are experiences only the patient can describe, such as nausea and pain. Objective data, or signs, are observable and measurable pieces of information, such as vital signs and lab results.
3. Components in a health history include biographical data, reason for health care visit, history of present illness, past medical and surgical history, family history, and lifestyle.
4. There are four methods of physical examination: inspection, palpation, percussion, and auscultation.
5. Some assessment findings in the older adult could include dry skin, loss of hair pigment, cataracts, decreased hearing, loss of teeth, increased blood pressure, decreased bowel sounds, decreased range of motion, stooped posture, and slower response to questions.
6. When assessing the pupils, use a penlight to observe the reaction to light, check for constriction or accommodation, and verify the presence of convergence.
7. Bradycardia exists when the heart rate is slow, usually below 60 beats per minute. Tachycardia is when the heart rate is fast, usually above 100 beats per minute.
8. The two types are objective and subjective. Neither is better than the other; they are both important in forming a fuller picture of the patient and his or her situation.
9. To evaluate mental status, ask the patient about a person, place, time, and situation. Also verify if they are alert and awake, lethargic, stuporous, or perhaps comatose.
10. To document accurately, write information down as soon as possible, be legible, organize the data, avoid judgments, record findings, use approved abbreviations, and be sure to be logical in the way the documentation flows.

## Apply What You Learned

1. Objective data can be seen, heard, touched, or smelled. Appearance of patient's clothes and overall hygiene can be considered objective.
2. Subjective data are experiences only the patient can describe. "Little joy in activities" and "loss of appetite" are subjective.
3. Initially, the nurse should focus the assessment on safety. Does the patient have plans to cause harm to himself or others? If not, maintain the focus on the patient's mental status. Due to the data presented, the patient may need a consultation with a mental health professional.

## Multiple Choice

| | | | |
|---|---|---|---|
| 1. | A | 9. | A |
| 2. | B | 10. | B |
| 3. | C | 11. | A |
| 4. | D | 12. | D |
| 5. | B | 13. | A |
| 6. | D | 14. | A |
| 7. | A | 15. | B |
| 8. | C | | |

## Chapter 6    Essential Nursing Pharmacology

## Key Terms

| | | | |
|---|---|---|---|
| 1. | B | 6. | F |
| 2. | J | 7. | C |
| 3. | D | 8. | H |
| 4. | A | 9. | E |
| 5. | G | 10. | I |

## Learning Outcomes

1. The six rights of medication administration are: right drug, patient, time, route, dose, and documentation.
2. Absorption is the first step in the passage of a drug through the body. It occurs from the time it enters the body until it reaches the bodily fluids that carry the drug to the site of action. Excretion is when the drugs are eliminated in the urine. The kidney is the most important organ of drug excretion.
3. The four names given to drugs are chemical, which includes the molecular structure of the drug; generic, which is the shorter version of the chemical name; trade, which is sometimes called the brand name and is usually trademarked or registered; and the official name, which is usually the trade name.
4. The purpose of a loading dose is to administer a higher-than-normal dose initially to quickly produce the desired result.
5. Idiosyncratic effects occur when a very small percentage of the population develops an unusual or unexpected response. Toxic effects occur when harmful, undesired effects or possibility of organ damage develop.
6. Agonists are drugs that combine with specific receptors to cause pharmacologic responses. Antagonists are drugs that prevent a receptor response or block normal cellular responses.
7. Polypharmacy is the use of many prescribed and over-the-counter drugs at the same time. This practice has been proven to be responsible for up to 30% of hospitalizations related to adverse medication reactions in older adults.
8. Age, body weight, genetics, ethnicity, disease conditions, and emotional state are some factors that affect drug responses.
9. Synergism is when two drugs are given together to cause a greater response than each one given separately, while potentiation is when the action of one drug increases the effect of the second drug.
10. Medication history components include the use of over-the-counter and herbal drugs, alcohol consumption, compliance with current medications, finances, allergies, liver or kidney disease, and cultural influences.

## Apply What You Learned

1. Educational points could include the importance of prescription drugs, various side effects associated with those drugs, and the importance of telling the physician about the over-the-counter drugs being taken in order to watch for interactions with the prescription drugs.
2. The nurse would point out the medication history to the physician in private prior to the physician going in to assess the patient so that the appropriate treatment can be prescribed.
3. Over-the-counter drugs are deemed safe for the general public. However, some over-the-counter drugs do not mix well with prescription medications, and this patient is mixing eight different types of medication, increasing the odds of an adverse reaction. This patient should be educated on all of his medications so that he can be involved in the treatment plan with his physician and feel some control over his health care plan.

## Multiple Choice

1. C
2. B
3. A
4. A
5. B
6. B
7. C
8. D
9. C
10. C
11. C
12. B
13. A
14. D
15. A

## Key Terms

1. I
2. H
3. C
4. E
5. J

6. F
7. G
8. D
9. A
10. B

## Learning Outcomes

1. ICF is within the cells; contains solutes such as electrolytes, glucose, and oxygen; and is essential for normal cell function. ECF is outside the cells and is distributed within three compartments: interstitial, intravascular, and transcellular.
2. Water in the body transports nutrients and oxygen to cells, takes waste such as carbon dioxide away from the cells, insulates and regulates body temperature, lubricates, and acts as a shock absorber.
3. Electrolytes help regulate water and acid–base balance, contribute to enzyme reactions, and are essential to neuromuscular activity.
4. Components of body fluid regulation are thirst, kidneys, the renin–angiotensin–aldosterone mechanism, antidiuretic hormone, and atrial natriuretic peptide.
5. Sweating, fever, draining wounds, urine, hemorrhage, and GI fluid loss can cause fluid volume deficits.
6. Renal failure, heart failure, medications, increased sodium intake, and cirrhosis of the liver are some causes of fluid volume excess.
7. Fluid status monitoring can be accomplished via assessing serum electrolytes, serum osmolality, hematocrit, urine specific gravity, and central venous pressure.
8. Isotonic solution is used to expand blood volume or replace abnormal loss; hypertonic solution is us to correct sodium depletion, replace water loss, and promote diuresis; and hypotonic solutions are u to maintain sodium and chloride levels as well as to replace water loss.
9. To reduce patients' risk for fluid imbalances, the nurse can monitor I&O, measure urine specific gravity, assess vital signs and peripheral pulses, take weight daily, provide oral fluids as ordered and monitor intake, and administer IV fluids as ordered.
10. Both hypo- and hyperkalemia affect cardiac function and can result in serious, even fatal, dysrhythmias.

## Apply What You Learned

1. The dietician would recommend high-potassium foods such as apricots, bananas, cantaloupe, spinach, meat, fish, and potatoes.
2. A consult for a thorough dental exam and perhaps a psychiatry consult based upon the statement regarding not eating solid foods. Ruling out a problem with broken or missing teeth and the diagnosis of anorexia nervosa would be necessary.
3. Potassium chloride because low chloride levels usually accompany low potassium. The physician may or may not order a vitamin supplement depending upon the results of lab tests, which will show any deficiencies.

## Multiple Choice

1. A
2. D
3. B
4. B
5. B
6. D
7. D
8. B

9. A
10. B
11. C
12. A
13. D
14. B
15. C

# Chapter 8    Caring for Patients in Pain

## Key Terms

1. E
2. J
3. F
4. A
5. H

6. I
7. D
8. B
9. C
10. G

## Learning Outcomes

1. Tolerance is the amount and duration of pain a person can stand before seeking relief. Threshold is the point at which each person recognizes pain.
2. Acute pain is temporary, has a sudden onset, and is localized. It usually lasts less than 6 months. Chronic pain is prolonged and lasts longer than 6 months. It is often unresponsive to conventional medical treatment.
3. Age, sociocultural background, emotional status, and past experiences with pain are factors that will affect the patient's response to pain.
4. It is a pump with a hand-held button that allows the patient to manage his or her own pain. The dose is programmed into the pump to prevent overdose. It helps the patient feel in control of pain relief.
5. Subjective data could include location, whether it radiates and where, superficial/deep, onset, pattern, quality, duration, aggravating and relieving factors, intensity, and method of relief.
6. Vital signs, skin moisture and color, dilated pupils, grimacing, guarding, restlessness, moaning, crying, being quiet, and being sad are possible objective indicators of pain.
7. Some misconceptions are that people who ask for opioids are usually addicts, it is best to wait until the patient has pain before giving medications, and opioids are too risky to be used to address chronic pain.
8. Interventions for chronic pain management include understanding the patient's expectations, including family, using the oral route (as this is long-term management), encouraging relaxation or distraction techniques, promoting rest and proper nutrition, and referring to a pain clinic.
9. Complementary therapy includes acupuncture, biofeedback, relaxation, distraction, hypnotism, and cutaneous stimulation.
10. Sedation, respiratory depression, constipation, and nausea are all possible side effects of opioids.

## Apply What You Learned

1. The nurse could ask the patient how she was directed to take the medication in order to verify that the patient understood the directions.
2. The patient might have a slow walk, be hunched over, grimacing, holding her back, and possibly moaning and sighing.
3. The patient could try deep breathing exercises, relaxation techniques, hypnosis, and distraction such as music.
4. Yes, because the medication bottle that had 30 pills was empty in only 14 days. Addiction is also a concern due to the information given by the patient regarding job status and overdue bills.

## Multiple Choice

1. A
2. D
3. A
4. B
5. C
6. A
7. B
8. B

9. B
10. C
11. D
12. D
13. B
14. C
15. D

## Chapter 9  Caring for Patients with Inflammation and Infection

### Matching

1. F
2. I
3. B
4. H
5. G

6. A
7. E
8. D
9. J
10. C

### Learning Outcomes

1. Inflammation can be caused by mechanical injuries; physical damage such as burns, poisons, bacteria or viruses; extreme heat or cold; hypersensitivity reactions; or by ischemic damage from a stroke or myocardial infarction.
2. There are three steps in the inflammatory response. They are the vascular response, during which blood flow to the injured area increases; cellular response, when white blood cells move into the injured area and ingest harmful bacteria; and healing and tissue repair, when normal structure and function begin to take place.
3. Local inflammation is manifested by redness, warmth, edema, pain, and loss of function.
4. Inflammation that is systemic will be manifested by fever, tachycardia, increased respirations, loss of appetite, fatigue, enlarged lymph nodes, and an elevated white cell count.
5. The chain of infection includes the microorganism, a reservoir, a portal of exit from the reservoir, a mode of transmission from the reservoir to the host, and an entry point into a susceptible host.
6. Chickenpox, gonorrhea, herpes simplex, lyme disease, rabies, tetanus, and tuberculosis are some common infectious diseases.
7. Risk factors for health care–associated (nosocomial) infections include chronic disease, history of frequent antibiotic use, invasive procedures, infections in other sites, burns, length of hospital stay, and the very young or very old age person.
8. Standard precautions involve hand washing, wearing clean gloves, changing gloves between patients, removing soiled clothing as soon as possible, cleaning spills with facility-recommended germicide, and using private rooms for patients when applicable.
9. Fever, sore throat, congestion, runny nose, nausea, weakness, pain on urination, malaise, joint pain, and diarrhea are some subjective data that may be present in the patient who has an infection.
10. Objective data for the patient with infection could include vital sign deviations, shortness of breath, altered mental status, dry mucous membranes, wheezing, enlarged lymph nodes, abnormal lab values, and decreased skin turgor.

### Apply What You Learned

1. The nurse should expect to see a urinalysis and a white blood cell count with a differential. There may be an order to culture the skin tear.
2. The patient does not answer questions appropriately and is confused, so it would be difficult to obtain accurate subjective data.
3. The nurse would expect a broad-spectrum antibiotic until test results are evaluated by the physician. There should also be an ointment for the skin tear as well as a dressing to maintain skin integrity and allow healing. Depending upon the facility's policy, a new Foley catheter might be placed after the resident is cleansed properly.

## Multiple Choice

1. A
2. C
3. B
4. A
5. D
6. D
7. D
8. B

9. A
10. C
11. D
12. C
13. A
14. B
15. A

## Chapter 10  Caring for Patients Having Surgery

## Matching

1. E
2. J
3. I
4. H
5. G

6. C
7. F
8. B
9. A
10. D

## Learning Outcomes

1. Inpatient surgery requires admission to a hospital before the procedure and nursing care in the hospital after the procedure; it may be planned or an unanticipated emergency situation. Ambulatory or outpatient surgery is performed on a patient who does not need inpatient nursing care. Procedure can be performed under local or general anesthesia, and the patient is able to return home following the procedure.

2. The perioperative nurse must have knowledge of surgical anatomy; anticipate functional disruptions related to surgery; know the potential consequences of disrupted function, risk factors, and potential complications; and understand the emotional and psychosocial effects of surgery on the patient and family.

3. Informed consent should include why the procedure is necessary related to the diagnosis, description and purpose of the procedure, possible benefits and risks, alternative treatments, risks if not done, physician advice to what is needed, and the right to refuse or withdraw the consent.

4. Preoperative care begins when the decision for surgery is made and ends when the patient is transferred to the surgical suite. The intraoperative phase begins with the patient's entry into the surgical suite and ends with transfer to the postanesthesia care unit. The postoperative phase begins when the patient is admitted to the PACU and ends when recovery from surgical intervention is complete.

5. The focus of preoperative care is to obtain informed consent, identify risk factors and needs, prepare the patient physically and psychologically, educate the patient and family, and discuss expected outcomes and recovery.

6. Nursing care on the day of surgery includes the following tasks: verify informed consent, complete skin prep as ordered, ensure ID bands are correct and in place, verify height and weight for anesthesia, remove hair pins and jewelry, obtain vital signs, and provide supportive care to patient and family.

7. Anesthesia is the use of chemical substances to produce a loss of sensation, reflex loss, or muscle relaxation during a surgical procedure with or without the loss of consciousness.

8. Hospital national patient safety goals include identifying patients correctly, improving staff communication, using medications safely, preventing infections, and preventing mistakes in surgery.

9. Dehiscence is a separation of an incision. The wound should be covered immediately with a sterile dressing moistened with normal saline and the surgeon notified. Evisceration is the protrusion of body organs from a wound dehiscence. Cover the wound with a moist sterile dressing or towels and notify the surgeon. Emergency surgery is necessary for repair.

10. Management of acute postoperative pain is of primary concern to the patient, surgeon, and nurse. Established, severe pain is more difficult to treat than pain that is at its onset. Initially, postoperative analgesics are administered at regular intervals or using patient-controlled analgesia (PCA). PC pumps help the patient to control pain and maintain therapeutic blood levels of pain medications. NSAIDs are administered to treat mild to moderate postoperative pain and as adjuncts to opioid analgesics. They should be given soon after surgery along with opioids unless contraindicated. Opioid analgesics are the foundation for managing moderate to severe postoperative pain.

## Apply What You Learned

1. The nurse would explain that PCA is a self-administration of opioid medications by a programmed infusion pump. It is utilized in the postoperative period for pain control and allows the patient to have some control over his or her care. It is programmed by the nurse to ensure safe dosages and locks out the patient once the dosage limit is reached.

2. Research has proven that severe pain is more difficult to treat than pain that is at its onset. Therefore, it is important for the patient to notify the nurse once he or she becomes uncomfortable in order to treat it effectively. If the pain is controlled, the need for opioids is lessened, or lower dosages will be required. Other pain medications may be utilized instead of an opioid if the patient reports pain at its onset.

3. The nurse would ask the patient about expectations about the pump and treatment, feelings concerning opioid medications such as morphine, concerns with addiction, and other methods of pain control. The nurse would also ask the patient about past experiences with pain and how he or she managed. The nurse would also show the patient how to use the pump and ask for a return demonstration, answering any patient questions as necessary.

## Multiple Choice

| | |
|---|---|
| 1. C | 9. C |
| 2. C | 10. C |
| 3. C | 11. C |
| 4. D | 12. B |
| 5. B | 13. B |
| 6. C | 14. C |
| 7. C | 15. B |
| 8. B | |

## Chapter 11    Caring for Patients with Altered Immunity

## Key Terms

| | |
|---|---|
| 1. E | 6. C |
| 2. G | 7. I |
| 3. B | 8. A |
| 4. F | 9. J |
| 5. D | 10. H |

## Learning Outcomes

1. Leukocytes are white blood cells involved in the immune system response. They start in the bone marrow and proceed to attack and destroy any foreign invaders at the site of involvement.

2. The immune system is composed of granulocytes, monocytes, and lymphocytes.

3. IgG is the most abundant immunoglobulin in the body and is active against bacteria, toxins, and viruses. It crosses the placenta to provide immune protection to the fetus. IgA provides local protection to prevent entry of bacteria and viruses, especially through the respiratory and gastrointestinal tracts.

4. Active immunity can be naturally acquired by actually developing the disease or artificially acquired through an immunization. Passive immunity involves injecting serum with ready-made antibodies from other humans or animals.

5. It is recommended that the adult be immunized for MMR, tetanus, hepatitis B, influenza, and pneumonia (older adults).

6. Anaphylaxis is an acute, immediate allergic reaction that requires immediate medical attention.

7. Hypersensitivity reactions can be immediate, cytotoxic, immune, or delayed.

8. Latex can be found in balloons, Band-Aids, condoms, Ace bandages, gloves, wound drains, stethoscopes, urinary catheters, and mattress covers.

9. An autoimmune disorder causes the immune system to mistake itself for nonself, and the body reacts against its own cells. Such disorders are more common in females and older adults and are frequently associated with a severe physical or psychological stressor.

10. Manifestations of HIV infection include fever, sore throat, headache, rash, fatigue, night sweats, weight loss, diarrhea, wasting syndrome, toxoplasmosis, herpes simplex/zoster, Kaposi sarcoma, and non-Hodgkin lymphoma.

## Apply What You Learned

1. The nurse would explain that KS is the most common cancer associated with HIV infection. Tumors develop in the lining of the small blood vessels, causing lesions on the skin. They start out painless but may become painful as the disease progresses.

2. The white patches in the mouth of this patient are called oral candidiasis or thrush. It is a fungal infection and may extend into the esophagus and stomach. It can produce an unpleasant taste in the mouth and can lead to painful swallowing.

3. Provide continuity of care and support to the patient and his partner. Balance activity with rest periods, provide a quiet room with minimal lighting, encourage socialization and pleasant conversation, focus on the things the patient can do and praise when tasks are accomplished, and provide distractions such as music, television, or movies.

## Multiple Choice

| | | | |
|---|---|---|---|
| 1. C | | 9. C | |
| 2. C | | 10. B | |
| 3. D | | 11. B | |
| 4. D | | 12. B | |
| 5. B | | 13. C | |
| 6. A | | 14. D | |
| 7. C | | 15. C | |
| 8. C | | | |

## Chapter 12    Caring for Patients with Cancer

## Key Terms

| | | | |
|---|---|---|---|
| 1. A | | 6. B | |
| 2. D | | 7. F | |
| 3. G | | 8. E | |
| 4. J | | 9. H | |
| 5. C | | 10. I | |

## Learning Outcomes

1. Benign neoplasms are localized growths with well-defined borders and are usually encapsulated. They tend to respond to body controls and once removed, they rarely recur. Malignant neoplasms grow aggressively and do not respond to body controls. They are not easy to remove and can recur. The term *cancer* refers to a malignant tumor.

2. An oncogene is a gene capable of promoting uncontrolled cellular growth. Carcinogens can "activate" the oncogene, thus allowing tumor development.

3. Controllable risk factors associated with cancer include stress, diet, weight, occupation, tobacco use, alcohol and drug use, and sun exposure.

4. HIV, hepatitis B, arsenic, asbestos, ultraviolet rays, radon, cigarettes, and hormones like estrogen are some carcinogens associated with cancer.

5. Possible cancer warning signs include persistent cough or hoarseness; unusual bleeding or discharge; recent unintended weight loss; recent change in a wart, mole, skin color, or texture; persistent functional change such as SOB; or a palpable lump in tissue.

6. There are many common manifestations of cancer. Pain, anemia, fatigue, bruising, anorexia, hoarseness, jaundice, constipation, and mental status changes, as well as difficulty swallowing, can be indicators of the disease.

7. Anorexia–cachexia syndrome is the effect of cancer cells on metabolism; cancer cells divert nutrition to their own use, inhibit food intake, and break down body tissue and muscle proteins to support their growth.

8. Tumors are classified and named by the tissue or cell of origin; adjectives are added to further specify the location. Other tumors are named for the discoverer of that particular cancer.

9. Superior vena cava syndrome, pericardial effusion, sepsis, spinal cord compression, and tumor lysis syndrome are oncologic emergencies.

10. Common side effects of chemotherapy are bone marrow suppression, nausea, vomiting, diarrhea, stomatitis, alopecia, and lethargy.

## Apply What You Learned

1. The nurse could encourage the patient to eat whatever is appealing in order to maintain caloric intake, even if it is not nutritionally sound. Encourage the intake of small, frequent meals with the use of an antiemetic. Nutritional supplements could be suggested, along with keeping a food diary to validate intake.

2. The nurse should begin by creating an open environment for the patient and family to discuss feelings realistically. Answer all questions honestly and encourage the patient to continue to take part in activities he enjoys.

3. Hospice services provide support and comfort for the patient and family, promoting their sense of control through the dying process. The hospice nurse is usually on call 24 hours a day and attends to the patient often. The nurse continually assesses the comfort of the patient to ensure he has as much pain control as possible. The nurse is often with the family when the patient dies. The support from the hospice is for the entire family, not just the patient.

## Multiple Choice

1. C
2. C
3. B
4. D
5. B
6. A
7. A
8. C
9. D
10. A
11. A
12. C
13. B
14. A
15. B

## Matching

| | | |
|---|---|---|
| 1. | H | 6. | B |
| 2. | E | 7. | D |
| 3. | A | 8. | F |
| 4. | C | 9. | I |
| 5. | G | 10. | J |

## Learning Outcomes

1. Palliative care is based on the principles of compassionate holistic caring, pain and symptom management, the facilitation of effective communication among health care team members, and provision of bereavement support. It is primarily planned and implemented to alleviate manifestations such as pain, nausea, dyspnea, confusion, anxiety, and depression. It is appropriate for patients in all disease stages.

2. Kübler-Ross identified the following stages of grief: denial, anger, bargaining, depression, and acceptance. She observed that not all people will go through the stages in order, and some may linger at a particular stage until they are ready to move on to the next stage. This staging process is individualized based upon the person's response to the loss.

3. Health, social status, possessions, lifestyle, sexual functioning, potential loss of body parts or functions, death, marital relationships, and reproduction are some common fears related to loss.

4. The types of advance directives are living will, durable power of attorney for health care, and durable power of attorney.

5. DNR, or no code, is written by the physician for the patient who is near death. This order is usually based on the wishes of the patient and family that no CPR be performed for respiratory or cardiac arrest. A comfort-measures-only order indicates that no further life-sustaining interventions are necessary and that the goal of care is a comfortable, dignified death.

6. As the patient's condition deteriorates, the nurse's knowledge of the patient and family guides the care provided. The nurse may provide opportunities for patients to express personal preferences about where they want to die and about funeral and burial arrangements. The nurse also encourages and supports the patient and family as they terminate relationships as a necessary part of the grief process. The nurse acknowledges this termination is painful and may stay with the patient and family at this time.

7. Manifestations of impending death include difficulty talking or swallowing, nausea or abdominal distension, urinary incontinence, constipation, decreased senses, weak or irregular pulse, decreasing blood pressure, decreased respirations, changes in level of consciousness, restlessness, and cyanosis of the extremities.

8. To maintain comfort of the dying patient, the nurse should maintain clean skin and bed linens. A draw sheet should be used to turn the patient frequently and comfortably. The nurse should provide gentle massage to promote circulation and shift edema as tolerated by the patient. Provide small, frequent sips of liquids. Provide oral care and clean secretions from eyes and nose. Administer ordered pain medications and oxygen.

9. Hospice care is for patients and their families when faced with a limited life expectancy. It is initiated for patients as they near the end of life and emphasizes quality rather than quantity of life.

10. Indications that death has occurred include absent respiration, pulse, and heartbeat; fixed, dilated pupils; release of stool and urine; pallor and waxen color; drop in body temperature; lack of reflexes; and flat encephalogram.

## Apply What You Learned

1. The type of care that this patient is to receive is termed *hospice*. It focuses on the quality of life that is left, not the quantity. The goal is to ensure a comfortable and dignified passing away.
2. When explaining procedures to this patient, the nurse needs to use short sentences, speak calmly yet loudly enough for them to hear, demonstrate by using touch in a sensitive and caring manner, and allow the patient to participate as much as possible. The nurse needs to ensure proper rest periods are offered during care, as the patient may tire easily.
3. The nurse would explain to the family that their loved one may not take in any more oral fluids or food items as the dying process begins. The patient may become agitated, which is common. The family needs to be reassured to not take this personally. Bowel and bladder incontinence is a common manifestation, and the staff will do everything possible to maintain clean and dry skin. The family will see skin color changes as the body proceeds in death. Vital signs will become irregular, and the level of consciousness will change. Aside from these findings, the nurse needs to be empathetic and open with the family. They will be looking to the nurse for emotional support during this confusing and difficult time.

## Multiple Choice

| | | | |
|---|---|---|---|
| 1. | B | 9. | B |
| 2. | D | 10. | C |
| 3. | A | 11. | B |
| 4. | A | 12. | C |
| 5. | C | 13. | B |
| 6. | C | 14. | A |
| 7. | B | 15. | B |
| 8. | C | | |

# Chapter 14 Caring for Patients Experiencing Shock, Trauma, or Disasters

## Matching

| | | | |
|---|---|---|---|
| 1. | H | 6. | E |
| 2. | B | 7. | A |
| 3. | J | 8. | G |
| 4. | C | 9. | D |
| 5. | I | 10. | F |

## Learning Outcomes

1. The five types of shock are: hypovolemic, anaphylactic, cardiogenic, septic, and neurogenic.
2. Compensatory, progressive, and irreversible are the three stages of shock. The compensatory stage occurs when decreased blood volume significantly reduces the heart's cardiac output. Blood pressure drops, and normal tissue perfusion cannot be maintained. At this point, the body initiates several mechanisms to maintain blood pressure and preserve vital organs. When the compensatory mechanisms fail, the progressive stage occurs. Without adequate tissue perfusion, the body's organ functions deteriorate. If the progressive stage is not treated rapidly, shock can progress to the irreversible stage, in which tissue and cellular death becomes so widespread that treatment cannot reverse the damage.
3. Common causes of hypovolemic shock are loss of blood volume as a result of trauma, surgery, GI bleeding, or hemophelia; internal fluid shifts as a result of cirrhosis with ascites, pleural effusion, pancreatitis, or intestinal obstruction; loss of body fluids through persistent and severe vomiting, diarrhea or continuous NG suctioning and massive diuresis from diuretics or diabetes insipidus; or loss of fluid through the skin as a result of profuse diaphoresis or burns.

4. Manifestations of anaphylactic shock are difficulty breathing, tachycardia, hypotension, restlessness, and a decreased level of consciousness.

5. An autotransfusion is the collection, filtration, and retransfusion of a patient's own blood. Blood from the chest cavity is the typical source for an autotransfusion.

6. Types of blood and blood products are whole blood, packed red cells, platelets, fresh frozen plasma, and cryoprecipitate.

7. Nursing implications for blood transfusions may be basic but are extremely important. Vital signs need to be obtained prior to transfusion so that there is a baseline record. The nurse must stay with the patient for the first 15 minutes of the transfusion to monitor for adverse reactions. Take and record vital signs during the transfusion as facility policy indicates. If a reaction occurs, stop the infusion, begin a drip of normal saline, and follow facility policy.

8. Trauma is any life-threatening occurrence, either accidental or intentional, that causes injuries. Leading causes of trauma are falls, motor vehicle crashes, and assaults. Trauma often kills or disables people during their most productive years of life.

9. Blunt trauma does not cause a break in the skin and can result in greater internal damage than what appears on the surface. A penetrating trauma results from foreign objects that pierce the body. Again, the external appearance does not determine the extent of internal damage.

10. Home safety tips include the following: use nonskid mats in the shower, install handrails by the tub and toilet as needed, use night-lights, turn pot handles away from the edge of the stove, keep a fire extinguisher near the stove, remove clutter from pathways, keep stairs well lit, install smoke alarms, and keep firearms unloaded and securely locked.

## Apply What You Learned

1. This would be classified as a blunt trauma injury because there is no break in the skin.

2. The nurse would ask what time the injury occurred, how fast was the ball going, where exactly on the head was he hit, did he lose consciousness, did he vomit, how his vision is now and how was it then, as well as about pain scale, radiating pain, stiffness in the neck, past traumas to the head, and complaints of dizziness and allergies. This information would help the nurse decide the urgency of the injury.

3. Radiography studies would be completed and could include CT scans, MRIs, and nuclear medicine. These studies would verify breaks, fractures, and fluid in the brain. Labs would also be drawn to check inflammatory response markers and to have a baseline should the patient experience complications. For treatment, the nurse would expect to provide a quiet and dimly lit room, ice packs for the first 24-hour period, pain medication as needed, neuro exam completed by the physician with follow-up by the nurse, and monitoring for nausea, vomiting, level of consciousness, and pain.

## Multiple Choice

1. D
2. B
3. A
4. D
5. C
6. B
7. A
8. A
9. D
10. A
11. B
12. D
13. B
14. C
15. D

## Matching

| | | | |
|---|---|---|---|
| 1. | H | 6. | F |
| 2. | B | 7. | I |
| 3. | J | 8. | E |
| 4. | G | 9. | D |
| 5. | C | 10. | A |

## Learning Outcomes

1. The heart is a hollow, cone-shaped organ approximately the size of an adult's fist. It weighs less than 1 pound. It is located behind the sternum and between the lungs in the thoracic cavity, slightly to the left of midline. The heart is a double pump. The right side receives blood from the body and pumps it to the lungs, and the left side receives blood from the lungs and pumps it to the body.

2. Diastole occurs when the ventricles fill and are relaxed. Systole occurs when the ventricles contract and eject blood into the pulmonary and systemic circuits.

3. The peripheral vascular system includes arteries, veins, and capillaries.

4. An electrocardiogram (ECG) is a record of the heart's electrical activity that is detected by electrodes placed on the skin. Patterns are used to detect dysrhythmias, myocardial damage or enlargement, and the effects of drugs.

5. Contractility is the natural ability of the cardiac muscle fibers to shorten during systole. It is necessary to move blood into circulation. With poor contractility, the blood does not move into circulation as necessary.

6. Cardiac output is the amount of blood pumped by the ventricles in one minute. It indicates how well the heart is functioning. The average adult cardiac output ranges from 4–8 liters per minute.

7. Activity level, autonomic nervous system, and hormones affect heart rate.

8. Components of a lipid profile include total cholesterol, triglycerides, high-density lipoproteins, low-density lipoproteins, and very low-density lipoproteins.

9. Doppler studies, transthoracic echocardiogram, stress tests, CXR, angiography, cardiac catheterization, CT, MRI, and radionuclear scans are used as diagnostic tools in cardiac dysfunction.

10. The purpose of a cardiac MRI is to show the thickness of the heart walls, size of the chambers, valve function, and coronary vessel flow.

## Apply What You Learned

1. Complete only a brief, focused assessment based on the acute symptoms. Notify the charge nurse and physician. Complete assessment data collection once the acute symptoms have been relieved and the patient is resting comfortably.

2. Diagnostic testing includes lipid profile, C-reactive protein, serum cardiac markers, cardiac hormones, 12-lead ECG, telemetry monitoring, and imaging studies.

## Multiple Choice

| | | | |
|---|---|---|---|
| 1. | A | 9. | D |
| 2. | C | 10. | C |
| 3. | C | 11. | B |
| 4. | B | 12. | A |
| 5. | D | 13. | B |
| 6. | C | 14. | A |
| 7. | A | 15. | B |
| 8. | A | | |

## Chapter 16   Caring for Patients with Coronary Heart Disease and Dysrhythmias

### Matching

| | | | |
|---|---|---|---|
| 1. | C | 6. | B |
| 2. | G | 7. | F |
| 3. | I | 8. | D |
| 4. | A | 9. | E |
| 5. | J | 10. | H |

### Learning Outcomes

1. Modifiable risk factors are hypertension, smoking, diabetes, obesity, inactivity, and a diet high in saturated fats. Nonmodifiable risk factors are age, gender, race, and heredity.

2. Atherosclerosis begins early in life. Lipids accumulate in the vessel wall. Vascular smooth muscle cells multiply, and scar tissue forms. These form a lesion that protrudes into the artery, eventually affecting blood flow. The surface of the plaque may become roughened or eroded. When this happens, platelets accumulate, and a blood clot forms. This clot may completely occlude the vessel.

3. Manifestations of angina include chest pain that may radiate to the neck, arms, shoulders, or jaw along with tight, squeezing, or heavy sensation. The patient may experience chest pain brought on by exercise, strong emotion, stress, cold, or heavy meals. The patient with angina also may have shortness of breath, pallor, anxiety, and/or fear.

4. Manifestations of an acute myocardial infarction include chest pain, tachycardia, shortness of breath, cool and clammy skin, diaphoresis, anxiety, feeling of impending doom, and nausea and vomiting.

5. Benign cardiac dysrhythmias can occur due to exercise or fear.

6. Cardioversion, also known as defibrillation, is used to treat rhythms that affect cardiac output and the patient's welfare. An electrical shock is administered to depolarize all cells of the heart at the same time. This often stops the abnormal rhythm and allows the sinus node to resume control of the rhythm.

7. Sudden cardiac death is when death occurs within one hour of the onset of cardiac symptoms.

8. Verapamil (Calan, Isoptin), diltiazem (Cardizem, Dilacor), and amlodipine (Norvasc) are calcium channel blockers.

9. PVCs are ectopic ventricular beats that occur before the next expected beat of the normal rhythm. They may be isolated or occur in patterns.

10. Atrial flutter is a very rapid and regular atrial rhythm. The patient usually complains of palpitations or a fluttering in the chest or throat.

### Apply What You Learned

1. The nurse needs to instruct the patient about pain management after the procedure. Movement of the affected arm and shoulder will be restricted for the first 24 hours. A chest x-ray will be done following the procedure for placement verification. The patient will receive a card with the pacemaker's name, model number, rate, and battery life. The patient needs to carry this card at all times and should wear a Medic-Alert bracelet. Teach the patient about the function of the pacemaker and how to take and record his pulse rate.

2. Decreased Cardiac Output, Risk for Ineffective Cardiac Tissue Perfusion, and Anxiety are nursing diagnoses related to this patient.

3. The patient should call his physician when the pulse rate is 5 or more beats per minute slower than the preset pacemaker rate, or if he experiences fever, dizziness, fainting, fatigue, weakness, chest pain, or palpitations. All of the patient's health care providers must be aware that the patient has a pacemaker implanted.

## Multiple Choice

| | | | |
|---|---|---|---|
| 1. B | | 9. B | |
| 2. C | | 10. B | |
| 3. B | | 11. C | |
| 4. C | | 12. D | |
| 5. D | | 13. B | |
| 6. D | | 14. B | |
| 7. B | | 15. C | |
| 8. A | | | |

## Chapter 17   Caring for Patients with Cardiac Disorders

## Matching

| | | | |
|---|---|---|---|
| 1. I | | 6. C | |
| 2. J | | 7. F | |
| 3. G | | 8. E | |
| 4. B | | 9. H | |
| 5. A | | 10. D | |

## Learning Outcomes

1. A: at high risk for heart failure but no current structural heart disease or symptoms, B: structural heart disease but no symptoms of heart failure, C: structural heart disease with current or prior symptoms of heart failure, and D: advanced heart disease with symptoms of heart failure at rest despite treatment.

2. Teaching points for the older adult include longer warm-up and cool-down with exercise, engaging in regular exercise 3–4 times a week, resting with feet elevated, maintaining adequate fluid intake, and reducing sodium intake in diet.

3. Although either side of the heart can fail, the left ventricle is affected more often than the right because of its high workload and oxygen demand. Left-sided heart failure results from ventricular muscle damage or overloading. As left ventricular function deteriorates, cardiac output falls. Impaired emptying of the left ventricle leads to increased pressure on the left side of the heart and in the pulmonary vascular system. Increased pressures in this normally low-pressure system push fluid from the blood vessels into interstitial tissues and the alveoli.

   The most common cause of right ventricular failure is left ventricular failure. Increased pressures in the pulmonary system or damage to the right ventricle impairs blood flow into the pulmonary circulation. The right ventricle and atrium become distended, and blood accumulates in the systemic venous system. Increased venous pressures lead to abdominal organ congestion and peripheral tissue edema.

4. Carditis can affect any layer of the heart in acute rheumatic fever; usually all three are involved. The valves become red and swollen, and small inflammatory lesions develop on the leaflets. As the inflammation resolves, scarring occurs, causing deformity. Rheumatic heart disease is slowly progressive valve deformity that can occur after acute or repeated attacks of rheumatic fever.

5. Laboratory testing helps establish the diagnosis of rheumatic fever. An echocardiogram is done to evaluate the structures and function of the heart. Management focuses on treating the primary infection, managing its manifestations, and preventing complications and recurrences of the disease. With acute carditis, treatment focuses on decreasing myocardial work. Antibiotics, NSAIDs, and corticosteroids may be ordered.

6. People with rheumatic heart disease, prosthetic heart valves, previous endocarditis, congenital heart conditions, and mitral valve prolapse should receive prophylactic antibiotics.

7. Pericarditis is inflammation of the pericardium, the outermost layer of the heart.

8. The types of heart murmurs are mitral stenosis, mitral regurgitation, aortic stenosis, and aortic regurgitation.

9. Cardiomyopathy is a disorder that affects the structure and function of the heart muscle.
10. MVP is a form of mitral insufficiency that occurs when the posterior cusp of the mitral valve flops back into the left atrium during systole. Most patients with MVP are asymptomatic and it is usually congenital in nature. It is commonly found in young women between the ages of 14 and 30.

## Apply What You Learned

1. This patient will have vital sign monitoring, neck vein distention and level of consciousness assessments, intake and output measurements, fluid restriction as ordered by the physician, oxygen and pulse oximetry, medications as ordered, and physical, emotional, and mental rest as needed.
2. The nurse would contact the dietician for a heart healthy diet and a social worker to assist in finding either home health care or a rehab facility where the patient can go until he is strong enough to manage on his own.
3. The nurse would teach the patient how to take his pulse before and after activities. The patient should also be encouraged to gradually increase activity and self-care as tolerated. The patient should be encouraged to ask for help when necessary because energy-saving techniques reduce cardiac workload.

## Multiple Choice

1. C
2. C
3. A
4. B
5. B
6. D
7. C
8. B
9. A
10. C
11. A
12. B
13. B
14. C
15. B

## Chapter 18    Caring for Patients with Peripheral Vascular Disorders

### Matching

1. B
2. J
3. E
4. I
5. C
6. F
7. G
8. A
9. D
10. H

### Learning Outcomes

1. (a) Isolated systolic hypertension is common. It develops as blood vessels become more rigid, decreasing their ability to expand and contract and increasing peripheral vascular resistance. (b) Chronic kidney disease is more common in older adults, contributing to hypertension. (c) The reflexes that maintain BP with position changes diminish, which can lead to a temporary fall in BP and an increased risk for falls and syncope.
2. Risk factors for hypertension include obesity, insulin resistance, excess alcohol consumption, smoking, physical stress, family history, age, and race.
3. Abdominal aortic aneurysms present with abdominal pain, lower back pain, cool and pale lower extremities, and a pulsating abdominal mass.
4. Marfan syndrome is a connective tissue disorder with three distinctive features: long, thin extremities, hyperextensible joints and other skeletal deformities; impaired vision; and cardiovascular defects, including MVP and weakness of the aorta. There is no cure for Marfan syndrome.

5. Arteriosclerosis is a common arterial disorder characterized by thickening, loss of elasticity, and calcification of arterial walls.
6. Complementary therapies for PVD include aromatherapy, healing touch, imagery, magnets, massage yoga, breathing exercises, and counseling.
7. Raynaud phenomenon is characterized by spasms of the small arteries and arterioles of the extremities. It is often secondary to another disorder and is sometimes called the red-white-and-blue disease. The spasms cause the fingers to go blue and white, and then red when the spasm is close to ending.
8. Risk factors for venous thrombosis include previous episodes, prolonged immobility, major surgery, myocardial infarction, certain cancers, pregnancy, childbirth, estrogen therapy, and obesity.
9. Varicose veins are irregular, tortuous veins with poorly functioning valves. They commonly affect the lower extremities.
10. Manifestations of varicose veins include severe, aching, leg pain; leg heaviness; itching of the leg; heat in the leg after prolonged standing, and visibly dilated veins in the leg.

## Apply What You Learned

1. The diagnosis most likely in this case is Raynaud phenomenon.
2. Treatments for this disease include smoking cessation, regular exercise, keeping the extremities warm by wearing gloves, and trying to avoid injury to the hands. Amputation is done only if blood flow cannot be restored and tissue necrosis has occurred.

## Multiple Choice

1. A
2. C
3. C
4. D
5. C
6. B
7. C
8. D
9. B
10. A
11. A
12. A
13. A
14. D
15. B

## Chapter 19    The Hematologic and Lymphatic Systems and Assessment

## Matching

1. C
2. D
3. G
4. B
5. H
6. J
7. F
8. E
9. I
10. A

## Learning Outcomes

1. Red blood cells, white blood cells, and platelets.
2. Hemoglobin is an oxygen-carrying protein that contains iron. This iron binds with oxygen and is synthesized within the RBC.
3. The differential includes neutrophils, eosinophils, basophils, lymphocytes, and monocytes.
4. Platelets are an essential part of the body's clotting mechanism. They are small fragments of cytoplasm without nuclei that contain many granules. They are stored in the spleen before being released into circulation. They live for approximately 10 days in circulating blood.

5. The lymphatic system assists the immune system by removing foreign matter, infectious organisms, and tumor cells from lymph. The largest lymphoid organ is the spleen, which filters the blood and produces lymphocytes and stores blood and platelets.

6. Lab tests used in lymphatic disorders are CBC, clotting studies, Coombs test, hemoglobin electrophoresis, and iron studies.

7. A bone marrow aspiration is done to analyze bone marrow and establish a diagnosis. Marrow is obtained from the posterior superior iliac crest, and the process may be painful for the patient despite the use of local anesthesia. The biopsy is done to examine for the presence of abnormal cells.

8. The five stages of hemostasis are vessel spasm, formation of the platelet plug, clot formation, clot retraction, and clot dissolution.

9. Blood transports oxygen, nutrients, and essential substances (such as hormones and other chemical messengers) to cells and tissues, and waste products away from tissues for removal from the body.

10. Normal hemoglobin is 13.5–18 g/dL for men and 12–15 g/dL for women.

## Apply What You Learned

1. In addition to a CBC that includes a WBC with differential, the nurse should expect a bone marrow aspiration to rule out malignancy.

2. Regarding the bone marrow aspiration, the patient should be informed that the procedure takes about 20 minutes. A local anesthetic will be used, but she may still feel some pressure with the procedure. It is important to remain very still during the procedure, and the site may ache for several days. The patient should be taught to report any unusual bleeding, drainage, or symptoms of infection immediately.

## Multiple Choice

| | | | |
|---|---|---|---|
| 1. | C | 9. | C |
| 2. | C | 10. | D |
| 3. | D | 11. | A |
| 4. | A | 12. | B |
| 5. | A | 13. | C |
| 6. | C | 14. | A |
| 7. | B | 15. | A |
| 8. | A | | |

## Chapter 20    Caring for Patients with Hematologic and Lymphatic Disorders

## Matching

| | | | |
|---|---|---|---|
| 1. | C | 6. | D |
| 2. | H | 7. | G |
| 3. | I | 8. | J |
| 4. | B | 9. | F |
| 5. | A | 10. | E |

## Learning Outcomes

1. Anemia reduces the oxygen-carrying capacity of the blood, leading to tissue hypoxia. As tissue oxygenation decreases, the body attempts to restore adequate oxygen delivery. The heart and respiratory rates increase. Blood is redistributed to vital organs, causing pallor of the skin, mucous membranes, nail beds, and conjunctiva. Tissue hypoxia may cause angina, fatigue, dyspnea on exertion, and night cramps. The kidneys release increased amounts or erythropoietin, which stimulates the bone marrow, causing bone pain. Poor oxygen delivery to the brain can cause headache, dizziness, and dim vision.

2. Thalassemia is an inherited disorder also caused by abnormal hemoglobin synthesis. It commonly affects people of Mediterranean, Asian, or African descent. The patient may have few symptoms or severe disease depending on the form of the disorder.

3. Asparagus, spinach, broccoli, green beans, corn flakes, oatmeal, and pasta contain folic acid.

4. Treatment for polycythemia focuses on reducing blood viscosity and volume and relieving symptoms.

5. Manifestations of leukemia include anemia, fatigue, tachycardia, malaise, lethargy, and dyspnea. The patient may also present with headache, altered level of consciousness, edema, anorexia, nausea, and bruising.

6. Leukemias are classified by their onset and duration (acute or chronic) and by the type of abnormal cells (myeloid or lymphocytic).

7. Nursing diagnoses related to leukemia include Risk for Infection, Impaired Oral Mucous Membranes, and Grieving.

8. Agranulocytosis is a decrease in granulocytes. Impaired WBC formation in the bone marrow is the usual cause.

9. Thrombocytopenia is a platelet count of less than 100,000 platelets per milliliter of blood. It is the most common cause of abnormal bleeding. It typically affects young adults from ages 20–40, and women more than men.

10. Risk factors associated with DIC are infection, malignancy, trauma, liver disease, hematologic disorders, venomous snakebites, and acute respiratory distress syndrome.

## Apply What You Learned

1. Hodgkin lymphoma would be the diagnosis.
2. Chemotherapy and radiation are the treatments of choice for this disease.
3. Nursing diagnoses for this disorder include Risk for Impaired Skin Integrity, Nausea, Fatigue, and Disturbed Body Image.

## Multiple Choice

1. A
2. D
3. D
4. C
5. C
6. C
7. B
8. B

9. A
10. D
11. A
12. C
13. C
14. C
15. A

## Chapter 21    The Respiratory System and Assessment

## Matching

1. I
2. E
3. H
4. D
5. J

6. A
7. B
8. F
9. G
10. C

## Learning Outcomes

1. The function of the upper respiratory system is to clean, humidify, and warm air. An open upper airway is needed for effective breathing.
2. The nose, sinuses, pharynx, and larynx are structures of the upper respiratory system.
3. The function of the lower respiratory system is to provide oxygen to the cells of the body and to eliminate carbon dioxide, a waste product of metabolism.
4. The lungs, bronchi, and alveoli are structures of the lower respiratory system.
5. Age-related changes in the respiratory system include decreased mobility of the rib cage, decrease in anterior–posterior diameter, weakening of respiratory muscles, and less effective cough and laryngeal reflexes.
6. Adventitious breath sounds are lung sounds that are abnormal.
7. Pulse oximetry is a noninvasive test used to evaluate and monitor oxygen saturation. The normal range is 95% or higher. The pulse oximeter sensor is usually applied to a fingertip, and the sensor emits infrared light to evaluate the oxygen saturation percentage. Infrared light is absorbed by hemoglobin.
8. In obtaining a throat swab, use a sterile cotton swab or throat swab kit. Identify the patient and purpose of the procedure and provide privacy. Have the patient in the seated position, if possible. Use Standard Precautions. Have the patient open his or her mouth, extend tongue, and say "ah." Quickly swab the tonsils, any exudate, and any red areas. Insert the swab into the specimen container and avoid contamination. Make sure to label the container and send to the laboratory.
9. The VP scan is used to detect pulmonary emboli, evaluate chronic lung disease, and assess the function of lung transplants.
10. Inform the family and the patient that the procedure takes 30–45 minutes. It may be done in the operating room, the patient's room, or a procedure room. The patient will receive an anesthetic and will have little discomfort. The patient may have a sore throat and hoarse voice following the procedure. The patient may have a fever for the first 24 hours after as well. The patient must report persistent cough, bloody sputum, wheezing, shortness of breath, or chest pain to the physician.

## Apply What You Learned

1. This patient will need a focused assessment of the respiratory system. Listening to the lungs in the front and the back will be important for the nurse to do.
2. Diagnostic testing the nurse might see include pulmonary function test (PFT), CBC, chemistries, throat cultures, and chest x-rays.
3. The nurse needs to ask the patient if there are factors that precipitate the symptoms and what alleviates them. The nurse should ask for remedies he may have tried at home along with asking what allergies he has. The nurse should also find out if the patient has traveled anywhere out of his region or has been exposed to something different in his environment.

## Multiple Choice

1. B
2. C
3. D
4. C
5. C
6. A
7. C
8. D
9. A
10. C
11. A
12. B
13. A
14. C
15. A

# Chapter 22  Caring for Patients with Upper Respiratory Disorders

## *Matching*

1. D
2. B
3. E
4. I
5. F

6. A
7. G
8. J
9. C
10. H

## *Learning Outcomes*

1. Viral pharyngitis is manifested by low-grade fevers, sore throat, headache, and a gradual onset. Patients with streptococcal infections will have a fever higher than 102°F, severe sore throat, patches on tonsils, malaise, and dysphagia.

2. Rhinitis, inflammation of the nasal cavities, is the most common upper respiratory disorder. Acute viral rhinitis is highly contagious. Most adults experience two to four colds each year. More than 200 strains of viruses can cause the common cold. These viruses are spread by hand-to-hand contact and by inhaling the virus. The virus can be spread to others for a few days before and after symptoms appear. Common manifestations of acute viral rhinitis are red, swollen, and congested nasal mucosa; clear, watery secretions with coryza; sneezing and coughing; low-grade fever; headache; malaise; and muscle ache. It can last from a few days to 2 weeks, is mild and self-limited, and secondary infections may follow.

   Manifestations of allergic rhinitis are pale, swollen, and congested nasal mucosa; thin, watery nasal discharge; itchy, watery eyes; sneezing; and headache. It occurs with exposure to allergens, and chronic congestion may cause snoring and postnasal drip.

   Influenza is a highly contagious viral respiratory disease that often occurs in epidemics. Yearly outbreaks affect about 48 million Americans each winter. The primary complication is bacterial pneumonia. Influenza viruses are transmitted by airborne droplet and direct contact. The incubation period is short, and the manifestations develop rapidly. Manifestations include coryza, sore throat, dry nonproductive cough that may become productive, substernal burning, chills and fever, headache, malaise, muscle aches, and fatigue and weakness. Fever and acute manifestations last up to a week; cough and fatigue may persist for several weeks.

3. All people over 6 months of age who do not have a contraindication to the vaccine should get it. It should not be given to people with an allergy to eggs.

4. To control URIs in long-term care: discourage people who are ill from visiting, provide tissues and masks to residents and visitors with symptoms, provide hand sanitizer and hand-washing supplies, ensure health care staff knows standard precautions, move residents with influenza symptoms to private rooms, and provide annual influenza vaccines to residents and staff.

5. Complementary therapies and practices are appropriate for treating many URIs. Herbal remedies such as echinacea and garlic have antiviral and antibiotic effects. Garlic supplements have been shown to reduce both the number and duration of URIs. Taken at the first sign of infection, echinacea may reduce the duration and symptoms of a common cold or influenza. Aromatherapy with essential oils can reduce congestion, enhance comfort, and promote recovery from a URI.

6. Ineffective Breathing Pattern, Ineffective Airway Clearance, and Disturbed Sleep Pattern are some nursing diagnoses for patients with URIs.

7. Also known as whooping cough, pertussis is an acute, highly contagious URI. Infants and young children have the highest incidence, but it also affects adults. The infected person should take prophylactic antibiotics.

8. Topical vasoconstrictors such as cocaine (0.5%), phenylephrine (1:1,000), or adrenaline (1:1,000) may be applied by nasal spray or on a cotton swab held against the bleeding site. The bleeding vessel may be cauterized using a chemical such as silver nitrate or Gelfoam.

9. Manifestations of nasal fractures include epistaxis, deformity or displacement, crepitus, soft tissue trauma, and instability of the nasal bridge.

10. Sleep apnea is the temporary absence of breathing during sleep. It affects men more than women. Obesity, enlarged tonsils, and the use of ETOH and sedatives before sleep contribute to sleep apnea. Obstructive sleep apnea is the most common form. It occurs when the pharynx is obstructed by the soft palate and tongue.

## Apply What You Learned

1. The nurse would tell the patient that his quality of life would be better if he were to quit drinking and smoking. Also, the healing process after surgery will be improved, and the risk of infection will be reduced. This patient may benefit from a support group such as AA or a psychologist to assist with the issue of terminal illness.

2. Encourage the family to visit whenever possible. Discuss postoperative communication techniques because this surgery will result in a loss of speech, and the patient will breathe through a permanent stoma in the neck. Teach the patient to cough and deep breathe effectively and to support the head when moving in bed. The patient and family should be taught how to protect the stoma from particulate matter in the air with gauze or another stoma protector. Encourage the patient and family to express their fears and anxieties.

3. Postoperatively, the nurse will be monitoring respiratory status and oxygen saturation, and will be maintaining humidified oxygen. The nurse will suction the tracheostomy using sterile technique as needed and provide care per protocol. The patient will be maintained on intravenous fluids and/or enteral feeding until he is able to take adequate amounts of food and fluids orally.

## Multiple Choice

1. C
2. B
3. B
4. C
5. C
6. D
7. B
8. C
9. C
10. D
11. B
12. D
13. D
14. B
15. A

## Chapter 23   Caring for Patients with Lower Respiratory Disorders

## Matching

1. C
2. E
3. A
4. J
5. B
6. F
7. H
8. D
9. I
10. G

## Learning Outcomes

1. Bronchitis is inflammation of the bronchi; emphysema is destruction of alveolar walls leading to large, abnormal air spaces in the lungs; and pneumonia is inflammation of the respiratory bronchioles and alveoli.

2. Aspiration of gastric contents into the lungs causes chemical and bacterial pneumonia. The risk for aspiration pneumonia is highest during emergency surgery and when cough and gag reflexes are depressed or swallowing is impaired.

3. Sputum gram stain and culture and sensitivity, CBC, WBC with differential, ABGs, pulse oximetry, chest x-ray, and bronchoscopy are some diagnostic testing to be done for pneumonia.

4. Ineffective Airway Clearance, Ineffective Breathing Pattern, and Activity Intolerance are nursing diagnoses for pneumonia.

5. TB is a chronic, recurrent infectious disease that usually affects the lungs. It can also involve other organs. Patients will present with fatigue, weight loss, anorexia, low-grade afternoon fever, and night sweats. The cough is dry initially and later becomes productive of purulent or blood-tinged sputum. This is when the patient usually seeks medical attention.

6. Less than 5 mm induration is negative for TB. Greater than 15 mm induration is positive for TB in all people, while 5–15mm induration can be positive for people with certain illnesses or risk factors.

7. Asthma attacks often can be prevented by avoiding allergens and other triggers. Modifying the home environment may help, pets may need to be removed from the household, and eliminating tobacco smoke in the house is important. For exercise-induced asthma, wearing a mask that retains humidity and warm air when exercising in cold weather may prevent an attack. Early treatment of respiratory infections is vital.

8. Manifestations of COPD include chronic cough (often productive of thick sputum), dyspnea, exercise intolerance, prolonged exhalation phase of breathing, barrel chest, distant breath sounds (possible wheezes and rhonchi), use of accessory muscles of respiration, possible cyanosis, and weight loss and tissue wasting.

9. Anterior–posterior chest diameter increases, taking on the appearance of a barrel. This occurs from the alveoli becoming less elastic and airways tending to collapse during exhalation. This causes air trapping in the lungs.

10. Lung cancer can present with endocrine symptoms (SIADH, Cushing syndrome), thrombophlebitis, cough, dyspnea, atelectasis, wheezing, and/or gynecomastia.

## Apply What You Learned

1. The patient will receive local anesthetic and may feel pressure upon insertion. Her breathing will improve once inserted. The nurse will document vital signs, breath sounds, saturation, color, and respiratory effort at least every four hours. The collection device will be kept below chest level and upright to maintain seal. The nurse will measure the drainage every 8 hours and report to the physician. If the tube is removed accidentally, the nurse will immediately apply a sterile, occlusive dressing and notify the physician.

2. Impaired Gas Exchange and Risk for Injury are nursing diagnoses that apply to this patient.

3. The nurse will frequently evaluate the respiratory status and oxygenation along with the amount of drainage and functioning of the drainage system. The nurse will document all teaching provided. The nurse will also document the patient's tolerance of ADLs, intake, output, and ambulation efforts.

## Multiple Choice

1. D
2. D
3. C
4. C
5. D
6. D
7. D
8. D

9. B
10. A
11. A
12. A
13. C
14. C
15. A

# Chapter 24   The Gastrointestinal System and Assessment

## Matching

| | | | |
|---|---|---|---|
| 1. | E | 6. | A |
| 2. | D | 7. | J |
| 3. | G | 8. | F |
| 4. | B | 9. | I |
| 5. | C | 10. | H |

## Learning Outcomes

1. Parietal, chief, mucous, and enteroendocrine cells.
2. The GI tract includes the mouth, pharynx, esophagus, stomach, small intestine, and large intestine.
3. The liver metabolizes carbohydrates, proteins, and fats. It eliminates old blood cells, cellular debris, and bacteria. The liver also stores blood, vitamins, and minerals, and excretes bile.
4. An upper endoscopy is used to evaluate swallowing problems, gastric reflux, and peptic ulcer disease.
5. The images can alert the physician to any obstruction or tumor that may be present.
6. Esophageal manometry measures the pressure of the esophageal sphincters and peristalsis. This tool can be helpful when the physician suspects swallowing dysfunction.
7. Liver, gallbladder, pylorus, duodenum, right adrenal gland, and a portion of the right kidney are located in the right upper quadrant of the abdomen.
8. The purpose of the stool specimen test for ova and parasites is to detect the presence of infective organisms.
9. When deficient in vitamins and minerals, the skin may be dry, flaky, and bruise easily. The patient may also have joint pain and peripheral neuropathies.
10. Weakness, weight loss, and increased heart rate are associated with water deficit. Increased blood pressure, weight gain, edema, and shortness of breath are indicators of water excess.

## Apply What You Learned

1. The nurse should ask the patient about recent lifestyle changes and weight loss. Find out if the patient has traveled out of the region or has noticed blood in his stool. The nurse should also find out what the pain is relieved by, exacerbated by, and if it radiates. The nurse should try to do a diet recall with the patient and explore what he has been eating over this time period.
2. Inspect, auscultate, percuss, palpate.
3. A CT scan will likely be done to rule out obstruction, along with a flat plate x-ray of the abdomen. Depending upon the results, the physician may order a barium enema or an upper endoscopy.
4. No, this patient should be NPO until diagnostic testing is complete and read by the physician.

## Multiple Choice

| | | | |
|---|---|---|---|
| 1. | A | 9. | D |
| 2. | C | 10. | A |
| 3. | C | 11. | D |
| 4. | B | 12. | B |
| 5. | D | 13. | C |
| 6. | D | 14. | C |
| 7. | B | 15. | B |
| 8. | C | | |

## Chapter 25 Caring for Patients with Nutritional and Upper Gastrointestinal Disorders

### *Matching*

| | | | |
|---|---|---|---|
| 1. | F | 6. | H |
| 2. | C | 7. | J |
| 3. | E | 8. | B |
| 4. | A | 9. | D |
| 5. | G | 10. | I |

### *Learning Outcomes*

1. Upper body obesity is identified by a waist/hip ratio greater than 1 in men and greater than 0.8 in women. In lower body obesity, the waist/hip ratio is less than 0.8. Lower body obesity carries a lower risk for complications than does upper body obesity.
2. Heart failure, hypertension, osteoarthritis, cancer, and muscle strains are some complications related to obesity.
3. Behavior strategies for weight loss include controlling the environment, controlling physical responses to food, controlling psychosocial responses to food, and making exercise a daily routine.
4. Aging, AIDS, burns, cancer, eating disorders, and surgery are conditions that are associated with malnutrition.
5. Catabolism is the breakdown of cells and tissues.
6. Enteral feedings may be used to meet all or part of the nutritional needs in patients who are unable to eat. Enteral feedings are done through various types of tubes that go directly into the GI tract via the nose, stomach, or jejunum.
7. Anorexia nervosa is an intense fear of weight gain and weight less than 85% of that expected for age and height.
8. Stomatitis is inflammation of the oral mucosa that affects eating.
9. Oral cancer can manifest as a sore in the mouth that does not heal; irregular white patches on the lips or tongue; erythroplakia; visible or palpable masses of the lips, cheek, or tongue; sore throat or a feeling of something caught in the throat; difficulty chewing, swallowing, or moving the jaw or tongue; asymmetry of the head, face, jaws, or neck; loosening of teeth, or dentures that no longer fit properly; swollen lymph nodes; and blood-tinged sputum.
10. GERD is the backward movement of gastric contents into the esophagus. It affects 15–20% of adults and is considered to be a common GI disorder.

### *Apply What You Learned*

1. For the surgery to be successful, the patient must be prepared for a complete change in lifestyle with regard to dietary habits. A strict diet will need to be followed for the rest of the patient's life to prevent weight gain and complications. The nurse must question the patient's readiness for the long-term behavioral changes that will accompany this procedure. The surgeon will then clarify the importance of following the diet, before obtaining the consent.
2. The patient needs to be instructed on the signs and symptoms of infection, dumping syndrome, postprandial hypoglycemia, and pernicious anemia.
3. Pain monitoring, airway monitoring, infection monitoring, nutrition monitoring, and ensuring accurate intake and output would be priorities regarding this patient.

## Multiple Choice

| | | | |
|---|---|---|---|
| 1. | C | 9. | B |
| 2. | D | 10. | A |
| 3. | B | 11. | C |
| 4. | B | 12. | C |
| 5. | A | 13. | B |
| 6. | B | 14. | B |
| 7. | C | 15. | D |
| 8. | C | | |

## Chapter 26    Caring for Patients with Bowel Disorders

### Matching

| | | | |
|---|---|---|---|
| 1. | E | 6. | B |
| 2. | A | 7. | D |
| 3. | C | 8. | G |
| 4. | F | 9. | J |
| 5. | I | 10. | H |

### Learning Outcomes

1. Diarrhea can result either from impaired water absorption or from increased water secretion into the bowel.
2. Dairy products, fruit juices, table sugar, coffee, and cola drinks can aggravate chronic diarrhea.
3. Older adults should be taught to increase dietary fiber to provide bulk and to drink six to eight glasses of water per day to assist in elimination. They should also remain as active as possible and not resist the urge to defecate when it is felt. The older adult should also be instructed about when to contact their primary care physician regarding changes in their bowel habits.
4. Saline, tap-water, soap-suds, phosphate, and oil-retention are types of enemas.
5. Irritable bowel syndrome is a motility disorder characterized by alternating periods of constipation and diarrhea.
6. Before a small bowel series, the patient may be restricted to a low-residue diet and receive a tap-water enema. The patient will be instructed to avoid food, fluids, and smoking for at least 8 hours before the exam. The patient needs to know that the test requires several hours to complete, and that barium is instilled through a weighted tube inserted into the small bowel. The patient should increase fluids after the test to expel the barium; stool will be chalky white for up to 72 hours after the exam due to the barium. The color will return to normal once the barium is excreted.
7. Malabsorption is ineffective intestinal absorption of nutrients. It usually occurs with disorders of the small intestine.
8. Manifestations of peritonitis include diffuse or localized pain, tenderness with rebound, board-like rigidity, diminished or absent bowel sounds, distention, nausea, fever, tachycardia, and restlessness.
9. Stool specimens, blood work, colonoscopies, and upper GI series with small bowel follow-through are some tests used to diagnose Crohn's disease.
10. Risk factors for colorectal cancer include over age over 50 years, family history, polyps of the rectum or colon, IBS, smoking, alcohol consumption, obesity, and a high-fat, low-fiber diet.

### Apply What You Learned

1. Nursing diagnoses for this patient would include Risk for Deficient Fluid Volume, Imbalanced Nutrition, Disturbed Body Image, and Diarrhea.

2. The information given is normal because the patient is slowly advancing her diet to prevent further irritations, has no present complaints of loose stools or pain, and the abdomen is slightly distended, which indicates that the inflammation is resolving. Her blood pressure is not a factor because it is within normal limits.

3. Along with dietary modifications, the patient should be instructed on stress reduction techniques. The patient should be taught about the short- and long-term effects regarding the illness. Discuss the increased risk for colorectal cancer and the need for medical follow-up.

## Multiple Choice

1. C
2. A
3. B
4. D
5. C
6. A
7. D
8. D

9. C
10. C
11. C
12. A
13. B
14. C
15. B

## Chapter 27 Caring for Patients with Gallbladder, Liver, and Pancreatic Disorders

## Matching

1. B
2. F
3. H
4. C
5. A

6. I
7. G
8. D
9. F
10. J

## Learning Outcomes

1. Presence of gallstones and alcoholism are risk factors for pancreatitis.
2. Biliary colic is a severe, steady pain in the right upper quadrant of the abdomen.
3. Some high-fat foods to avoid in cholelithiasis are whole milk products, deep-fried foods, bacon, gravies, most nuts, chocolate, and snack foods such as potato chips.
4. Hepatitis is an inflammation of the liver. It is usually caused by a virus but also may be caused by alcohol, toxins, or gallbladder disease. It can be acute or chronic in nature. Some types of hepatitis include A, B, C, delta, and E.
5. Jaundice can develop when excess RBCs are destroyed and the liver is unable to process all the released bilirubin, when damaged liver cells are not able to metabolize and excrete bilirubin, or when bile is obstructed within the biliary system and thus bilirubin excretion is impaired.
6. Injection drug users, people on hemodialysis, recipients of clotting factors, male prison inmates, patients and staff of institutions for the developmentally disabled, high-risk populations (Alaska Natives, Pacific Islanders, and immigrants from HBV-endemic areas), household members and partners of HBV carriers, international travelers to HBV-endemic areas, recipients of certain blood products (such as clotting factors) and people at risk for sexual transmission should be vaccinated for hepatitis B.
7. In cirrhosis, functional liver cells are destroyed, disrupting the metabolic functions of the liver. Lost cells are replaced by scar tissue that forms constrictive bands within liver lobules and disrupts blood flow within the liver. Impaired blood flow leads to portal hypertension and ultimately to liver failure.
8. Diagnostic testing for cirrhosis includes CBC, liver function tests, blood chemistries, coagulation studies, ultrasound, liver biopsy, and an upper endoscopy.

9. In acute pancreatitis, the patient presents with severe epigastric pain that may radiate to the back. The patient may have nausea, vomiting, decreased bowel sounds, tachycardia, cool skin, elevated WBCs, and low magnesium. Chronic pancreatitis will present with elevated glucose levels, elevated amylase and lipase, constipation, anorexia, vomiting, weight loss, and persistent episodes of upper abdominal pain radiating to the back.

10. Lab tests for pancreatic disorders include serum amylase, serum lipase, urine amylase, serum calcium, serum magnesium, white blood cells, and carcinoembryonic antigen.

## Apply What You Learned

1. Nursing interventions for this patient will include checking daily weight before breakfast, organizing dietician consult, assessing mental status, measuring abdominal girth every shift, taking bleeding precautions, keeping head of bed elevated and legs elevated as tolerated, and utilizing home health for follow-up.

2. The nurse needs to assess the ability and willingness of the wife to help with food preparation, follow-up medical care, and family responsibilities. Support groups such as Alcoholics Anonymous should be suggested. The wife should be made aware of social services and home health agencies that can offer assistance. The wife must also be aware of the discharge instructions set forth by the physician so that she can help her husband understand the treatment plan. The wife needs to understand the prognosis of the illness so as to provide the best care and quality of life to her husband.

3. Excess Fluid Volume, Imbalanced Nutrition, Disturbed Thought Processes, and Ineffective Protection are some nursing diagnoses related to this patient.

## Multiple Choice

1. D
2. A
3. D
4. B
5. D
6. C
7. A
8. B
9. C
10. C
11. D
12. A
13. D
14. B
15. A

## Chapter 28 The Urinary System and Assessment

## Matching

1. D
2. C
3. F
4. B
5. E
6. H
7. G
8. A
9. I
10. J

## Learning Outcomes

1. Nephrons are the functional units of the kidneys. Each kidney contains at least 1 million nephrons, which process blood to make urine.

2. The ureters move urine from the kidney to the bladder using peristaltic waves. The ureters contain smooth muscle and are innervated by the autonomic nervous system. They are bilateral tubes that are about 10–12 inches long.

3. Glomerular filtration is a passive process in which fluid and solutes move from the blood in the glomerulus into Bowman's capsule. The amount of fluid filtered from the blood into the capsule per minute is called the glomerular filtration rate.

4. Normal GFR in adults is 120–125 mL/min.

5. Dysuria is painful urination, nocturia is urinating more than once during the night, and hematuria is blood in the urine.

6. Lab tests used are BUN, serum creatinine, creatinine clearance, and serum albumin.

7. Uroflowmetry is used to evaluate voiding and function of the lower urinary tract. It generally is used to evaluate retention and incontinence. It is noninvasive and measures the volume and rate of urine flow.

8. The 24-hour urine specimen is urine that is saved in a container for a 24-hour period. All urine must be collected, or the test must be restarted. The specimen is kept in the refrigerator or on ice. At start time, urine from the first void is discarded. Notes should be placed in the patient's bathroom, over the bed, on the chart, and in the Kardex so that all persons know the test is in progress. Appropriate documentation regarding the specimen must be complete.

9. Inform the patient and family that the procedure takes about 30–45 minutes and that local or general anesthesia may be used. The patient may feel pressure or an urge to urinate as the scope is inserted. Burning on urination for a day or two after the procedure is considered normal. The patient will need to notify the physician if the urine remains bloody, if there is bright red bleeding, or if the patient has a fever or flank pain. Increasing fluids will decrease pain and difficulty with urination and reduce the risk of infection.

10. Components involved in urine studies are urinalysis, culture and sensitivity, 24-hour urine tests, electrolytes, protein, and creatinine.

## Apply What You Learned

1. For a 24-hour urine test, verify the physician's order, obtain a specimen container with preservative (if indicated). Label with identifying data, the test, time started, and time of completion. Post notices or chart, Kardex, on the door, over the bed, over the toilet, and alert all personnel that all urine is to be saved. At start time, have patient empty bladder completely and discard urine. Save and refrigerate or keep on ice all urine for the next 24 hours. At the end of collection, have patient empty the bladder one last time and save this urine in the container. Take entire specimen container with requisition to the lab. Chart appropriately. Remember that if one urine is missed, the test must be restarted.

2. A CT may be done to visualize structures of the urinary tract. A renal scan may be done to evaluate blood vessels and perfusion of the kidneys and ureters. Also, an ultrasound may be done to examine the size, shape, and position of the bladder and kidneys.

3. The physician is going to evaluate the status of sodium, chloride, potassium, calcium, and magnesium in the blood. Creatinine and protein will be evaluated also to help identify kidney disease.

## Multiple Choice

1. C
2. C
3. B
4. D
5. C
6. C
7. A
8. B
9. C
10. A
11. B
12. C
13. D
14. A
15. A

# Chapter 29   Caring for Patients with Kidney and Urinary Tract Disorders

## Matching

1. C
2. A
3. G
4. H
5. I

6. B
7. J
8. D
9. E
10. F

## Learning Outcomes

1. Urinary incontinence is involuntary urination. It is common among older adults.
2. The types of incontinences are stress, urge, voiding difficulties, reflex, and functional.
3. Older adults with UTIs may be asymptomatic or may present with nocturia, incontinence, confusion, behavior changes, lethargy, anorexia, or "just not feeling right."
4. Azotemia is an increased blood level of nitrogenous waste, including urea and creatinine.
5. Manifestations of urinary stones include dull, aching flank pain; nausea and vomiting; cool, clammy skin; and pain radiating to suprapubic region, groin, scrotum, or labia.
6. Goose, organ meats, sardines, herring, venison, chicken, crab, pork, salmon, and veal are all high in purines.
7. Impaired Urinary Elimination, Risk for Impaired Skin Integrity, and Disturbed Body Image are nursing diagnoses related to bladder cancer.
8. Complications related to dialysis include both systemic and fistula complications. Hypotension is the most frequent complication occurring during hemodialysis. Muscle cramps are also common. Bleeding may occur due to altered clotting and the use of heparin during dialysis. Infection is a significant risk. AV fistula problems include infection and clotting or thrombosis, which may cause fistula failure and require development of a new site. This failure can result in depression and an altered self-concept.
9. Renal failure is a condition in which the kidneys are unable to remove accumulated waste products from the blood. It may be acute or chronic, and lead to fluid and electrolyte imbalance.
10. Maintain accurate I&O records, weigh the patient daily, document vital signs at least every 4 hours, frequently assess heart and breath sounds, place in Fowler's position, restrict fluids as ordered, administer medications with meals, turn frequently, provide good skin care, administer diuretics as ordered, and monitor serum electrolytes as ordered.

## Apply What You Learned

1. The nurse would explain that the kidneys are no longer able to remove waste products from the blood. If the cause is known, explain that to the patient and family in lay terms. The dialysis will be done to remove the waste products that the kidneys no longer can. The dialysis will act as the "filter." To ensure understanding, ask the patient for a return demonstration on information given and correct them when necessary. Keeping the patient and family informed will lead to a better outcome and improved cooperation.
2. The patient's blood is pumped to a dialyzing unit, where it moves past a semipermeable membrane. A solution, dialysate, is warmed to body temperature and passed along the other side of the membrane. Solutes diffuse through the membrane and into the dialysate. Excess water is removed from the blood by creating a higher fluid pressure on the blood side of the membrane.
3. Excess Fluid Volume, Imbalanced Nutrition, Risk for Infection, and Disturbed Body Image are nursing diagnoses that pertain to this patient.

## Multiple Choice

| | | | |
|---|---|---|---|
| 1. | C | 9. | A |
| 2. | B | 10. | A |
| 3. | B | 11. | A |
| 4. | A | 12. | C |
| 5. | C | 13. | A |
| 6. | C | 14. | C |
| 7. | D | 15. | B |
| 8. | D | | |

## Chapter 30   The Reproductive System and Assessment

## Matching

| | | | |
|---|---|---|---|
| 1. | I | 6. | G |
| 2. | B | 7. | H |
| 3. | D | 8. | F |
| 4. | J | 9. | E |
| 5. | A | 10. | C |

## Learning Outcomes

1. The reproductive system in men includes the paired testes, the scrotum, ducts, glans, and penis.
2. The internal structures of the female reproductive system include the ovaries, fallopian tubes, uterus, and vagina.
3. The ovaries produce estrogens, progesterone, and androgens.
4. Mammography is used to screen for breast cancer in women who have no symptoms. It can detect tumors that are too small to be detected by a clinical breast exam or breast self-exam.
5. Pelvic ultrasound is used to identify tumors and to monitor ovulation in women. Abdominal and vaginal approaches are used. For the vaginal approach, the transducer is covered with a condom and coated with transducer gel.
6. Transrectal ultrasonography is used on men to assess the prostate gland, urethra, seminal vesicles, and vas deferens. It may also be used to guide a needle biopsy of the prostate. It is sometimes performed under sedation.
7. The prostate gland is the size of a walnut and encircles the urethra just below the urinary bladder. Secretions of the prostate gland make up about one-third of the volume in semen.
8. The ovarian cycle has three phases. The follicular phase lasts from the 1st to the 10th day of the cycle. The ovulatory phase lasts from the 11th to the 14th day, ending with ovulation, and the luteal phase lasts from the 14th to the 28th day.
9. Spermatogenesis is sperm production. It begins with puberty and continues throughout a man's life, with approximately 500 million sperm produced daily. Spermatogenesis takes 64 to 72 days.
10. Seminal fluid is made of secretions from the seminal vesicles, the epididymis, prostate gland, and Cowper's gland. It nourishes the sperm, provides volume to the semen, and increases its alkalinity.

## Apply What You Learned

1. The menstrual cycle, or ovarian cycle, has three phases and lasts 28 days. Days 1–10 are the follicular phase that involve the primary, secondary, and vesicular follicles. Ovulation occurs in the next phase and lasts from the 11th to the 14th day. This is the time when a woman is the most fertile. The luteal phase lasts from the 14th day to the 28th day, sets up the corpus luteum, and degenerates the corpus luteum. This is when the period occurs.

2. The first thing the nurse needs to do is provide as much privacy as possible. Then initiate friendly dialogue so that trust can be achieved. Then the nurse can ask the teen what she knows and believes to be true about menstruation. The interview process may take place with or without a parent/guardian present. A parent is usually present for a physical exam.

## Multiple Choice

1. C
2. D
3. B
4. A
5. C
6. D
7. C
8. A
9. B
10. D
11. D
12. A
13. B
14. C
15. A

## Chapter 31    Caring for Male Patients with Reproductive System Disorders

## Matching

1. D
2. A
3. E
4. C
5. G
6. J
7. H
8. B
9. I
10. F

## Learning Outcomes

1. Benign prostatic hyperplasia develops only in men who have testes. Testosterone is converted to dihydrotestosterone (DHT) in the prostate gland and stimulates growth of the prostate. Although testosterone levels decrease with aging, estrogen levels increase. Estrogen appears to make the prostate more responsive to DHT, promoting its growth. Increases in estrogen levels in relation to testosterone levels may contribute to BPH. BPH develops as small nodules that form and grow in the central and transition zones of the prostate, next to the urethra. The expanding prostate compresses surrounding tissue, narrowing the urethra.

2. Manifestations of prostate cancer include reduced urinary stream, increased frequency, erectile dysfunction, bone or joint pain, back pain, lower extremity weakness, weight loss, fatigue, anemia, and bowel or bladder dysfunction.

3. Digital rectal exam (DRE) is a screening tool to identify an enlarged prostate. The lab will run serum PSA levels and possibly test a tissue sample. The physician may also order imaging studies such as a CT or MRI to identify possible tumors.

4. Radiation therapy may be used to treat prostate cancer, delivered by either external beam or implants of radioactive seeds. Radiation therapy may also be used to reduce the size of bone metastasis, control pain, and restore function in patients with advanced prostate cancer. Following surgery for testicular cancer, radiation therapy is used to treat cancer in the retroperitoneal lymph nodes. It can also be used to help treat cancer of the penis.

5. Robotic-assisted laparoscopic prostatectomy (RALP) is the most commonly used procedure, through which the prostate is removed through a laparoscope. In addition, there are three types of open radical prostatectomy (ORP). With retropubic prostatectomy, the prostate gland is removed through an abdominal incision and the bladder is left intact. In a suprapubic prostatectomy, the prostate gland is removed through an abdominal incision into the bladder. With a perineal prostatectomy, the prostate gland is removed through a perineal incision between the scrotum and anus.

6. Impaired Urinary Elimination, Risk for Incontinence, Sexual Dysfunction, and Pain are nursing diagnoses for prostate dysfunction.

7. Testicular torsion is a twisting of the testes and spermatic cord, and is a potential medical emergency Boys and young men up to age 20 are at greatest risk for testicular torsion; the cause is unclear.

8. It is important to teach the patient how to perform a testicular self-examination. The nurse should emphasize the importance of regular exams and teach the patient that persistent undescended testicles should be reported to the physician.

9. Testicular cancer is the most common cancer in men between the ages of 15 and 35. It is one of the most treatable, with a cure rate of greater than 90%. The cause is unknown, but risk factors can include a family history, undescended testicles, race, and ethnicity. Beginning at age 15, all men should perform monthly testicular self-exams to assess for lumps or irregularities. Testicular cancer grows within the testicle and eventually replaces most of the normal tissue. Usually only one testicle is affected.

10. Diagnostic tests related to ED are done to help identify the cause of the problem and include blood tests such as a chemistry profile and testosterone, prolactin, thyroxine, and PSA levels to identify systemic disorders that may be causing the dysfunction; nocturnal penile tumescence and rigidity (NPTR) to monitor erections that occur during REM sleep; and cavernosometry and cavernosography to evaluate blood flow to and from the penis.

## Apply What You Learned

1. This patient will have labs done to evaluate the PSA level. The physician may also order a CT or MRI to evaluate the nodule for size, shape, and location. A urinalysis will also be ordered to rule out infection and calculi.

2. This patient is a candidate for a prostatectomy. In this procedure, the prostate gland will be removed and the bladder will be left intact. The patient will have an indwelling catheter postprocedure to allow appropriate healing.

3. The nurse will talk to the patient about possible stress incontinence after the catheter is removed. Postoperative complications such as infection will need to be discussed so that the patient and his partner know when to notify the physician. The nurse needs to reinforce follow-up care to monitor the disease and the healing process.

## Multiple Choice

| | | | |
|---|---|---|---|
| 1. | D | 9. | B |
| 2. | B | 10. | D |
| 3. | A | 11. | B |
| 4. | B | 12. | B |
| 5. | A | 13. | C |
| 6. | C | 14. | A |
| 7. | A | 15. | D |
| 8. | A | | |

## Chapter 32   Caring for Female Patients with Reproductive System Disorders

## Matching

| | | | |
|---|---|---|---|
| 1. | C | 6. | H |
| 2. | D | 7. | J |
| 3. | F | 8. | G |
| 4. | A | 9. | B |
| 5. | E | 10. | I |

## Learning Outcomes

1. Several complementary therapies can be used to help relieve perimenopausal symptoms. Black cohosh is used as an estrogen enhancer; chasteberry for hormone balancing; St. John's wort for mood changes; motherwort for palpitations and hot flashes; skullcap for anxiety; and dong quai for an estrogen enhancement. Hypnotherapy, meditation, and homeotherapy are also used. Massage and aromatherapy massage are also effective.

2. HRT is often used to relieve unpleasant manifestations of menopause and reduce some of the risks associated with estrogen deficiency. HRT relieves hot flashes and night sweats, and decreases vaginal dryness. Perineal tissue atrophy, which can lead to painful intercourse and urinary incontinence, can also be relieved with HRT.

3. PMS is a symptom complex of irritability, depression, edema, and breast tenderness preceding menses. It is a common disorder, and the pathophysiology is not clearly understood, though hormonal changes are thought to contribute to the problem.

4. A hysterectomy is a removal of the uterus. The ovaries are usually left in place unless other conditions warrant their removal.

5. Endometriosis is a common condition in which endometrial tissue is found outside the uterus. Endometrial tissue may be found on the ovary and other pelvic organs or tissues, and rarely in other organs such as the lungs. The cause is unknown, but it may be caused by backflow of menstrual blood carrying endometrial cells through the fallopian tubes into the pelvis.

6. Diagnostic testing used regarding ovarian cysts include LH, FSH and serum testosterone, glucose tolerance tests, and a laparoscopy.

7. Vaginitis is an inflammation or infection of the vagina. Such infections are common and may be fungal, protozoal, or bacterial.

8. PID is an infection of the pelvic organs. It is usually caused by infection with *Neisseria gonorrhoeae* and/or *Chlamydia trachomatis*. Patients with PID are often infected with more than one organism. It is a major cause of infertility. It usually affects young, sexually active women who have multiple partners.

9. Cervical cancer is common. Early detection and intervention have substantially reduced the incidence of invasive cervical cancer as well as the number of deaths due to cervical cancer. Most occurrences are related to infection of the cervix with human papillomavirus (HPV). Other risk factors for cervical cancer include early sexual experience, multiple sex partners, HIV infection, unprotected sex, smoking, and a poor diet. Early cancer causes no symptoms. With progression, the woman may notice pain in the back or thighs, hematuria, bloody stools, anemia, and weight loss.

10. Uterine prolapse is caused by stretching of the ligaments that normally support the uterus within the pelvis. Increased pressure within the abdomen also can lead to uterine prolapse.

## Apply What You Learned

1. This patient's risk factors are nipple discharge, breast pain, skin rash, and family history.

2. Mammograms, ultrasounds, CT, MRI, cytologic exams, and tissue biopsy are diagnostic tests done to confirm breast cancer.

3. Nursing diagnoses include Decisional Conflict regarding treatment options, Grieving, Risk for Infection, Risk for Injury, and Risk for Disturbed Body Image.

4. During the grieving process, the nurse must listen attentively to expressions of loss and observe for nonverbal cues. The nurse must also spend time with the patient and not rush interactions. The nurse needs to explain that periods of depression, anger, and denial are normal and expected. The nurse needs to locate community resources and ensure that the patient has support from family.

## Multiple Choice

| | | | |
|---|---|---|---|
| 1. D | | 9. D | |
| 2. B | | 10. C | |
| 3. D | | 11. B | |
| 4. A | | 12. B | |
| 5. C | | 13. A | |
| 6. A | | 14. B | |
| 7. C | | 15. A | |
| 8. A | | | |

## Chapter 33    Caring for Patients with Sexually Transmitted Infections

### Matching

| | | | |
|---|---|---|---|
| 1. G | | 6. D | |
| 2. I | | 7. B | |
| 3. C | | 8. A | |
| 4. E | | 9. F | |
| 5. J | | 10. H | |

### Learning Outcomes

1. Health care workers are at risk for contracting some STIs from their patients through unprotected contact with infected blood and body fluids. Infants can be infected by their mothers *in utero* or during delivery. Children can be infected through incest of sexual abuse. Victims of sexual assault are also at risk. People with multiple sexual partners have the highest risk of acquiring an STI. The incidence also high in people of color in urban settings with lower socioeconomic status and less education. T... incidence of STIs is highest among young people.

2. Risk factors for STIs include personal history or partner history of STI, teen sexual activity, use of oral contraceptives, unprotected sex, multiple sex partners, and pregnancy.

3. Chlamydial infections are thought to be the most common STI and the leading cause of pelvic inflammatory disease. *Chlamydia trachomatis* is a bacterium that behaves like a virus, reproducing only within the host cell. It is spread by any sexual contact. It is asymptomatic in most women until it has invaded the uterus and uterine tubes. Men are also asymptomatic and eventually can present with urethral discharge.

4. Females with gonorrhea are often asymptomatic but may have vaginal discharge, abnormal menses, and dysuria. Men may have dysuria, increased urinary frequency, and purulent urethral discharge.

5. Some nursing diagnoses related to STIs include Ineffective Health Maintenance, Impaired Skin Integrity, Risk for Injury, Anxiety, Situational Low Self-Esteem, Sexual Dysfunction, and Impaired Social Interaction.

6. The best preventative measure against STIs is abstinence. However, when there is concern about preventing STIs, it is important to know that the more sexual partners one has, the greater the risk of contracting an STI. Use condoms, vaginal spermicides, and lubricants with each sexual encounter. Seek out a physician if you suspect an STI, and go back for follow-up care. Do not have sex until you and your partners are completely cleared to do so by a physician.

7. Genital herpes is a chronic and often asymptomatic STI. Currently, no cure is available for genital herpes. It is spread by vaginal, anal, or oral–genital contact. It has an incubation period of 3 to 7 days. Within a week of exposure, painful red papules appear in the genital area.

8. Syphilis, if not treated, can lead to blindness, paralysis, mental illness, cardiovascular damage, and death. Penicillin has significantly reduced the incidence of syphilis. Syphilis often occurs with one or more other STIs, such as HIV or chlamydia. It begins with an ulcer at the site of inoculation that may become a rash, especially on the palms of the hands or soles of the feet. Mucous patches may appear in the oral cavity along with a sore throat. Flu-like symptoms may also be present. The latent stage of syphilis can last up to 50 years. During this stage, no symptoms are apparent and it is not transmissible by sexual contact. It can be transmitted through blood, however.

9. Females may be asymptomatic or may have frothy, excessive vaginal discharge, erythema, edema, and pruritus. Males usually are asymptomatic also, though they may have urethritis, penile lesions, or inflammation.

10. Reportable STIs include syphilis, gonorrhea, and AIDS. Chlamydia is reportable in most but not all states.

## Apply What You Learned

1. The student nurse can create an environment in which the teens feel respected and safe to discuss concerns about the disease and its effect on the teens' lives. Providing privacy and confidentiality along with compassionate communication are key with this age group. The student nurse must also be nonjudgmental and supportive while informing the teens that an STI is not a punishment but a consequence of sexual behavior.

2. Subjective assessment data include current symptoms, general health, past medical history, sexual activity and measures used to prevent pregnancy and infection, possibility of pregnancy and last menstrual period, and substance use such as tobacco, alcohol, or other drugs. Objective data include vital signs; inspect skin, mucous membranes of mouth and oropharynx, abdomen for contour and visible peristalsis, and genitalia (including the penis, external urinary meatus, scrotum, and anus in men and the perineum, labia majora, labia minora, vaginal opening, and anus in women); auscultate bowel sounds; and palpate abdomen and suprapubic region for tenderness and inguinal lymph nodes for swelling or tenderness.

3. The student nurse will inform the teens that risk factors for STIs include pregnancy, multiple sexual partners, unprotected sexual activity, and a history of STIs.

## Multiple Choice

| | | | |
|---|---|---|---|
| 1. | A | 9. | B |
| 2. | C | 10. | D |
| 3. | D | 11. | D |
| 4. | D | 12. | D |
| 5. | D | 13. | D |
| 6. | A | 14. | A |
| 7. | D | 15. | B |
| 8. | A | | |

## Chapter 34   The Endocrine System and Assessment

## Matching

| | | | |
|---|---|---|---|
| 1. | C | 6. | F |
| 2. | G | 7. | H |
| 3. | D | 8. | J |
| 4. | E | 9. | B |
| 5. | A | 10. | I |

## Learning Outcomes

1. The primary function of the endocrine system is to regulate the body's internal environment. This regulation is maintained through the function of various hormones within the endocrine system. T hormones regulate growth, reproduction, metabolism, and fluid/electrolyte balance.
2. TSH, T3, T4, growth hormone, serum Ca, serum phosphate, HbA1c, and blood glucose, as well as urine tests for glucose and ketones, can be ordered to diagnose an endocrine disorder.
3. An MRI uses a super magnet and radio frequency signals to elicit a response from hydrogen nuclei. As a result, tumors of the pituitary gland and hypothalamus can be identified.
4. The thyroid gland increases metabolic rates and lowers serum calcium levels. It is shaped like a butterfly and sits on either side of the trachea.
5. The hypothalmus controls the anterior pituitary function by regulating temperature, fluid volume, and growth. It also responds to pain, pleasure, hunger, and thirst stimuli.
6. The pancreas is the primary organ involved in diabetes. It is located behind the stomach between the spleen and duodenum. It serves two major functions. Acini cells secrete digestive enzymes into the duodenum, and the islets of Langerhans release insulin and glucagon into the bloodstream.
7. Insulin's primary function is to regulate blood glucose levels. Insulin release increases when blood glucose levels rise and decreases when blood glucose levels fall. When a person eats food, insulin levels rise in minutes, peak in 30–60 minutes, and return to baseline in 2–3 hours.
8. Exophthalmos is forward protrusion of the eyeballs. It is diagnosed upon physical examination for some endocrine disorders.
9. The patient must fast during the test and drink 75 grams of glucose. This test determines the level of glucose 2 hours after drinking the 75 grams. Levels should return to normal, but a level higher than 200 mg/dL indicates diabetes.
10. The adrenal cortex stimulates gluconeogenesis and increases blood glucose levels. It also regulates blood volume and electrolytes.

## Apply What You Learned

1. and 2.  Growth hormone promotes growth of body tissues. Thyroid-stimulating hormone stimulates secretion of thyroid hormone. Adrenocorticotropic hormone stimulates the adrenal cortex to secrete glucocorticoids. Melanocyte-stimulating hormone controls pigmentation of the skin. Follicle-stimulating hormone stimulates ovary development and egg and sperm production. Luteinizing hormone stimulates ovulation and secretion of sex hormones in males and females. Prolactin stimulates breast milk production.

## Multiple Choice

| | | | |
|---|---|---|---|
| 1. | C | 9. | D |
| 2. | B | 10. | D |
| 3. | C | 11. | A |
| 4. | A | 12. | D |
| 5. | D | 13. | C |
| 6. | B | 14. | A |
| 7. | C | 15. | B |
| 8. | B | | |

## Chapter 35    Caring for Patients with Endocrine Disorders

### Matching

1. D
2. C
3. B
4. G
5. H

6. E
7. A
8. F
9. J
10. I

### Learning Outcomes

1. Diabetes insipidus is a condition that results from antidiuretic hormone insufficiency. There are two types: neurogenic and nephrogenic. The patient will present with extreme thirst, polyuria, weakness, and dehydration.

2. A thyroid storm is an extreme state of hyperthyroidism that is rare today. This disorder may result from untreated hyperthyroid, infection, diabetic ketoacidosis, physical/emotional trauma, or thyroid surgery. It is life threatening and requires immediate medical attention.

3. A goiter is an enlargement due to iodine deficiency, most commonly seen on the neck.

4. The patient with myxedema coma will present with seizures, lethargy that quickly progresses to a coma, and hypothermia. This is a life-threatening emergency.

5. The nurse caring for a patient having a subtotal thyroidectomy will provide standard preoperative care and give ordered antithyroid medications and iodine preparations before the surgery. Following the surgery, the nurse will provide standard postoperative care, place the patient in a semi-Fowler's position and support the head and neck with pillows; and monitor and report the following complications to the physician—hemorrhage, respiratory distress, laryngeal nerve damage, tetany, and thyroid storm.

6. Cushing syndrome is a chronic disorder in which the adrenal cortex produces excessive amounts of the hormone cortisol. It is more common in women between the ages of 30 and 50.

7. The patient with Addison disease will present with bronzing over the knuckles, knees, and elbows. Muscle weakness, irregular pulse, lethargy, depression, anorexia, and salt cravings may also be present.

8. Nursing diagnoses for endocrine disorders could include Disturbed Thought Processes, Hypothermia, Constipation, Activity Intolerance, and Risk for Impaired Skin Integrity.

9. Pheochromocytoma is a benign tumor of the adrenal medulla. The tumor produces excessive amounts of epinephrine and stimulates the sympathetic nervous system.

10. Corticosteroids are the main medication class for the treatment of Addison disease. Examples are prednisone, methylprednisolone, and dexamethasone.

### Apply What You Learned

1. Tests for this patient would include T3, T4, TSH levels along with a routine CBC and CMP.

2. The diagnosis of hypothyroidism would be made due to the manifestations of weight gain, loss of appetite, and always being cold.

3. Levothyroxine is one of the most common medications used in the treatment of hypothyroidism. Patient education regarding body changes, dietary modifications, and rest periods will be part of the treatment plan.

## Multiple Choice

| | |
|---|---|
| 1. B | 9. C |
| 2. C | 10. B |
| 3. B | 11. A |
| 4. A | 12. B |
| 5. C | 13. A |
| 6. B | 14. C |
| 7. B | 15. A |
| 8. A | |

## Chapter 36    Caring for Patients with Diabetes Mellitus

### Matching

| | |
|---|---|
| 1. F | 6. G |
| 2. B | 7. J |
| 3. E | 8. A |
| 4. I | 9. C |
| 5. H | 10. D |

### Learning Outcomes

1. Type 1 diabetes is a state of absolute insulin deficiency. It usually occurs before childhood, and the patient is prone to developing ketoacidosis. These patients are insulin dependent. Type 2 is a state of sufficient insulin to prevent ketoacidosis but insufficient to lower blood glucose levels. It usually occurs after the age of 30, and most patients are obese. They are not insulin dependent but may requir insulin.

2. Polyuria, polydipsia, polyphagia, weight loss, fatigue, and malaise are some manifestations of type 1 diabetes.

3. Glycosuria is excess glucose in the urine.

4. The four types of insulin are rapid-acting, short-acting, intermediate-acting, and long-acting.

5. Long-acting insulin, such as Lantus, has an onset of 2 hours, the peak is not defined, and the duration of this medication is 24 hours.

6. When administering insulin, be sure to discard any vial whose expiration date has passed. Be sure to check the patient's blood glucose 30 minutes before giving insulin and check type and dose with another nurse. Keep a record of blood glucose levels and monitor for signs and symptoms of hyper- and hypoglycemia.

7. Patients should be instructed to maintain caloric intake to coincide with their body weight. Artificial sweeteners such as Sweet & Low and Nutrasweet should be used instead of pure sugar. Patients with diabetes should be taught to have 15–20% of their daily caloric intake in protein and have 20–35 grams of fiber daily. They should be taught to limit alcohol and have less than 7% of their daily calories from saturated fats.

8. Ketonuria is a presence of ketones in the urine, which usually occurs when the blood glucose is greater than 250 mg/dL.

9. When a patient is in a hyperosmolar hyperglycemic state, he or she will present with severely elevated blood glucose levels, extreme dehydration, and an altered level of consciousness.

10. Peripheral vascular disease may present with loss of hair on lower legs, shininess of the skin, cold feet, thick toenails, diminished pulses, pain at rest, and intermittent claudication.

## Apply What You Learned

1. The nurse should request a dietary consult with a diabetes education specialist. The nurse should also provide examples of sugar substitutes, proteins, and fiber-rich foods. The patient should be taught to order out in moderation, and to add fruits and vegetables as snacks. The nurse should instruct the patient on staying well hydrated by drinking water, especially when the patient wants a sugary snack. Ensure that the dietician can provide real-world examples of food at work that will suit his lifestyle.

2. This patient will receive insulin by injection to cover the 312 mg/dL blood glucose reading. Monitoring and documentation should be completed regarding urine output and other signs and symptoms of hyperglycemia. The nurse should monitor for signs of altered levels of consciousness and visual disturbances. A recheck of the blood glucose should be done according to facility policy or as the physician requests.

3. The patient needs to be educated on the importance of keeping the feet clean and dry, especially in between the toes. The feet should be inspected daily for cracks in the skin and other breaks in skin integrity. The nurse should instruct the patient to never go barefoot and to always wear appropriately fitting shoes and cotton or wool socks. The patient should be taught to cut toenails after washing because they will be softer, and to cut them straight across to avoid ingrown toenails. The physician will inspect the feet upon each follow-up visit, so let the patient know that he will be asked to remove his socks and shoes.

## Multiple Choice

1. A
2. B
3. C
4. A
5. A
6. C
7. D
8. D
9. A
10. C
11. A
12. A
13. C
14. C
15. A

## Chapter 37   The Nervous System and Assessment

## Matching

1. D
2. C
3. B
4. I
5. G
6. J
7. E
8. H
9. A
10. F

## Learning Outcomes

1. The myelin sheath is a white fatty substance that protects and insulates axons.
2. The three layers of meninges are dura mater, arachnoid, and pia mater.
3. The cerebellum is connected to the midbrain, pons, and medulla. Like the cerebrum, it has two hemispheres. It coordinates involuntary muscle activity and fine motor movements, as well as balance and posture.
4. A reflex is an involuntary motor response to a stimulus.

5. The ANS is part of the peripheral nervous system. It is responsible for maintaining the body's internal homeostasis. It regulates respiration, heart rate, digestion, urinary excretion, body temperature, and sexual function.
6. The primary function of the eye is to convert patterns of light from the environment into a message that is transmitted via the optic nerve to the brain. The brain gives meaning to the message, allowing us to make sense of what we see.
7. Age-related changes in vision include decreased corneal sensation and tear secretion, constriction of the pupil, decreased elasticity and increased density of the lens, loss of rods at the periphery of the retina, and loss of fat and subcutaneous tissue around the eyes.
8. The primary functions of the ear are hearing and maintaining balance.
9. The 10th cranial nerve is the vagus nerve. It is responsible for the function of swallowing, controls heart and respiratory rates and digestion, and controls the sensation in pharynx and larynx.
10. Focused assessment of the patient with a neurologic disorder begins with identifying the patient's LOC. When the patient's LOC is altered, the nurse may need to ask the family for information. In addition, respiratory status, numbness, tingling, tremors, problems with coordination or balance, loss of movement in any part of the body, or difficulty walking or using the hands will be assessed. The nurse needs to determine when symptoms first began and whether they are constant or intermittent. The nurse determines if the patient has difficult with speaking, seeing, hearing, tasting, or detecting odors. The nurse also assesses the patient's memory, feelings of anxiety or depression, recent changes in sleep patterns, ability to perform ADLs, sexual activity, and weight changes. The nurse will ask about medications the patient is taking as well as about past medical history and family health history. The patient will also be assessed for occupational exposure to toxic chemicals or materials, use of protective headgear, and the amount of time doing repetitive motion tasks. The nurse will also assess diet and use of alcohol, tobacco, or recreational drugs.

## Apply What You Learned

1. Cranial nerves IX and X are involved with swallowing.
2. The cranial nerves related to eyeball movement are III, IV, and VI.

## Multiple Choice

| | | | |
|---|---|---|---|
| 1. | D | 9. | B |
| 2. | A | 10. | C |
| 3. | B | 11. | D |
| 4. | C | 12. | A |
| 5. | B | 13. | A |
| 6. | C | 14. | B |
| 7. | D | 15. | B |
| 8. | B | | |

## Chapter 38    Caring for Patients with Intracranial Disorders

## Matching

| | | | |
|---|---|---|---|
| 1. | I | 6. | C |
| 2. | J | 7. | A |
| 3. | E | 8. | G |
| 4. | B | 9. | D |
| 5. | H | 10. | F |

## Learning Outcomes

1. Risk for Ineffective Tissue Perfusion: Cerebral; Ineffective Breathing Pattern; Risk for Imbalanced Nutrition: Less Than Body Requirements; Risk for Impaired Skin Integrity; Impaired Physical Mobility; and Risk for Infection.

2. Manifestations of concussion include immediate loss of consciousness for less than 5 minutes, drowsiness, confusion, dizziness, headache, and blurred or double vision.

3. The three types of hematomas related to the brain are epidural, subdural, and intracerebral.

4. Someone with an altered level of consciousness may be disoriented to person, place, and time. The person may have a short attention span and poor memory, or may appear restless, agitated, and combative.

5. Brain tumors are abnormal growths within the cranium. Their cause is unknown, but prolonged exposure to certain chemicals and radiation increases the incidence.

6. Manifestations related to brain tumors include personality changes, inappropriate behavior, impaired judgment, recent memory loss, motor deficits, expressive aphasia, seizures, headache, and visual deficits.

7. Manifestations of CVAs are the motor deficits hemiplegia, hemiparesis, and facial droop; the speech deficits aphasia and dysarthria; the visual deficits diplopia and homonymous hemianopia; the sensory–perceptual deficits agnosia, apraxia, and neglect syndrome; and the cognitive and behaviour changes memory loss, short attention span, poor judgment, poor problem-solving ability, emotional lability, and depression.

8. A seizure is a brief disruption of brain function caused by abnormal electrical activity in the nerve cells of the brain. It may occur as an isolated event or as part of a disorder.

9. Initial treatment focuses on controlling the seizure. Long-term management involves identifying the cause and preventing future seizures. Collaborative care includes diagnostic testing, medications, and, in some cases, surgery.

10. Meningitis is an inflammation of the meninges of the brain and spinal cord. Once bacteria or virus enter the CNS, an inflammatory response begins in the meninges, CSF, and ventricles. Recovery is usually uneventful.

## Apply What You Learned

1. The likely diagnosis for this patient is CVA.

2. Diagnostic tests that the nurse would expect to see ordered include CT scan, MRI, cerebral arteriography, Doppler ultrasound, PET, and lumbar puncture.

3. The treatment plan for this patient will include antiplatelet medications such as Plavix. Low-dose aspirin taken daily may also be utilized. If there are residual effects from the CVA, the patient may require physical, occupational, or speech therapies. He may need to perform the therapy in a long-term care facility or rehabilitation center.

## Multiple Choice

| | | | |
|---|---|---|---|
| 1. | B | 9. | D |
| 2. | B | 10. | B |
| 3. | D | 11. | A |
| 4. | C | 12. | D |
| 5. | D | 13. | C |
| 6. | C | 14. | B |
| 7. | A | 15. | C |
| 8. | B | | |

# Chapter 39 Caring for Patients with Degenerative Neurologic and Spinal Cord Disorders

## Matching

1. D
2. J
3. E
4. I
5. C
6. G
7. A
8. B
9. F
10. H

## Learning Outcomes

1. Myasthenia gravis is a chronic autoimmune disorder affecting women under 40 and men older than 60 years of age. Patients experience periods of exacerbations and remissions. Stress, pregnancy, and secondary infections may trigger an acute onset. For unknown reasons, the thymus gland produces antibodies that block or reduce the number of acetylcholine receptors at each neuromuscular junction. Nerve impulses cannot be sent to the cranial nerves that control muscles of the face, lips, tongue, neck, and throat. This causes weakness of the facial, speech, and chewing muscles.

2. Bell palsy (facial paralysis) is associated with the herpes simplex virus. Inflammation causes edema and pressure on the facial nerve, resulting in necrosis. This leads to sudden weakness and paralysis on one side of the face. There is also pain around or behind the ear. Most patients improve within a few weeks to months, although some are left with residual paralysis.

3. The purpose of plasmapheresis is to remove T lymphocytes that cause inflammation.

4. Manifestations related to Parkinson disease include tremors; rigidity of the neck, shoulders, and trunk; bradykinesia; drooling; excess sweating on face and neck; oily skin; memory loss; and inability to initiate voluntary movements.

5. Huntington disease is a progressive, inherited neurologic disease. There is no cure, and each child who has a parent with HD has a 50% chance of inheriting the disease. It involves a lack of a neurotransmitter, GABA, and eventually leads to personality changes, intellectual changes, and movement dysfunction.

6. ALS, commonly known as Lou Gehrig disease, involves loss of motor neurons in the spinal cord and brainstem. When these impulses cannot be sent to the brain, they lose strength and atrophy. Although body function decreases, the person remains mentally alert.

7. Rabies is a viral infection of the CNS caused by an animal bite.

8. Spinal cord injuries are usually due to trauma. The spinal cord provides a two-way path to conduct impulses between the brain and body. Spinal cord injury mechanisms include hyperflexion, hyperextension, and cord compression. Most injuries occur in the lumbar and cervical regions, where the vertebrae are not protected by other parts of the skeleton, such as the rib cage or pelvis.

9. Autonomic dysreflexia is an exaggerated sympathetic response in patients with SCIs at or above the T6 level. The patient develops a pounding headache; bradycardia; blurred vision; flushed, diaphoretic skin above the lesion and pale, cold, dry skin below it; goose bumps; and anxiety.

10. Spinal cord tumors may be primary or secondary, benign, or malignant. Most of them occur in the thoracic and cervical areas. They compress the cord, spinal nerve roots, and surrounding blood vessels. Pain is often the first sign and is described as localized or radiating.

## Apply What You Learned

1. Discuss the following topics with the patient and family: avoiding stress, extreme heat or cold, and physical overexertion; medications and side effects; bowel and bladder schedule; ways to prevent complications such as pressure ulcers; ways to cope with pain; the importance of follow-up care; and community agencies that are available as the disease progresses.

2. The student nurse should encourage the patient and family to express their feelings. Seek out a counselor if needed. Refer them to a support group and provide information about the National MS Society. Also refer them to state vocational rehabilitation agencies as needed.

## Multiple Choice

| | | | |
|---|---|---|---|
| 1. | A | 9. | C |
| 2. | B | 10. | A |
| 3. | C | 11. | C |
| 4. | B | 12. | B |
| 5. | A | 13. | D |
| 6. | B | 14. | A |
| 7. | B | 15. | D |
| 8. | B | | |

## Chapter 40    Caring for Patients With Eye and Ear Disorders

### Matching

| | | | |
|---|---|---|---|
| 1. | D | 6. | B |
| 2. | G | 7. | H |
| 3. | A | 8. | J |
| 4. | C | 9. | F |
| 5. | E | 10. | I |

### Learning Outcomes

1. Manifestations of conjunctivitis include redness, itching, tearing, and discharge of the eye.
2. Cataracts are the clouding of the lens of the eye that impairs vision. They are common, and most people over 65 years of age have some cataracts. A cataract usually affects both eyes, but each eye tends to develop at a different rate. As a cataract matures, both near and distance vision are affected. Details become obscured and light rays become scattered, causing a problem with glare and adjusting between light and dark environments.
3. Manifestations of glaucoma include gradual loss of peripheral vision, blurred vision, halos around lights, difficulty focusing on near objects, possible nausea and vomiting, clouded cornea, and fixed pupils.
4. Face the patient, so that the two of you are seated about 2 feet apart. Instruct the patient to cover the right eye and focus on your face. Cover your left eye and focus on the patient's face. Midway between the patient and yourself, bring a light-colored object into the field of vision from the side. Ask the patient to indicate when the object is seen. Check all visual fields of both eyes in this manner.
5. The retina can remain intact but separate from the choroid or tear and fold back on itself. A break or tear in the retina allows fluid to seep between the retina and choroid, separating these layers. If the layers remain separated, the neurons of the retina become ischemic and die, causing permanent vision loss. For this reason, retinal detachment is a medical emergency that requires prompt treatment.
6. Macular degeneration is a common cause of blindness in older adults. With aging, the neurons of the macula may atrophy or separate from the choroid. When the macula is damaged, central vision becomes blurred and distorted, but peripheral vision remains intact. It usually affects activities such as reading and sewing.
7. To prevent external otitis, stay out of the water for 7–10 days or until completely healed, use earplugs to keep cold water out of ears, use a hair dryer on the lowest setting to dry ear canals after swimming, and do not insert cotton swabs or any other object into the ear canals.
8. Tinnitus is ringing in the ears.
9. Vertigo is a sensation of whirling or movement when there is none and is the key symptom of inner ear disorders.
10. Disturbed Sensory Perception, Impaired Verbal Communication, and Social Isolation are nursing diagnoses related to hearing loss.

## Apply What You Learned

1. The nurse needs to orient the patient to his environment verbally and physically. Describe items within the area such as chairs, steps, and carpeting. Give the patient verbal cues when he is performing a task so that he feels empowered to continue. Keep hallways and rooms free of clutter when the patient is ambulating.

2. The family can orient the patient as to the position of the food on the plate. Using the face of a clock is familiar to use as a reference. For example, carrots are at 3 o'clock. Juice is at 12. This way, the patient maintains independence and nutrition.

3. There are state, local, and national agencies to help coordinate services for people with impaired vision.

## Multiple Choice

1. C
2. C
3. C
4. A
5. A
6. D
7. D
8. B
9. C
10. C
11. B
12. B
13. A
14. A
15. C

# Chapter 41   The Musculoskeletal System and Assessment

## Matching

1. F
2. E
3. J
4. I
5. C
6. H
7. A
8. B
9. G
10. D

## Learning Outcomes

1. Ligaments are bands of connective tissue that connect bones to bones.

2. Three types of muscle tissue are skeletal, smooth, and cardiac.

3. Adduction is to move toward the midline of the body, and abduction is to move away from the midline of the body.

4. Long bones, such as those in the arms and legs, have a shaft, called a diaphysis, and two broad ends, called epiphyses. Short bones include those of the wrist and ankle. Flat bones, including skull bones, the sternum, and ribs, are thin and flat; most are curved. Irregular bones vary in size and shape. They include the vertebrae, the scapulae, and the bones of the pelvis.

5. ESR is the erythrocyte sedimentation rate, which is a nonspecific measure of inflammation.

6. Testing for calcium is important for monitoring the skeletal system because most of the body's calcium is in the bones and teeth. Adequate total body calcium is vital to maintain bone mass. Blood levels increase when calcium is released from the bone.

7. Bone absorptiometry is a test used to diagnose osteoporosis by measuring bone mineral density. Special x-ray imaging techniques are used to expose the patient to very low amounts of radiation and help predict fracture risk by comparing the individual's bone mass to that of a healthy 25- to 35-year-old person.

8. Arthroscopy uses a flexible fiberoptic endoscope to view joint structures and tissues. It is used to identify torn tendons or ligaments, an injured meniscus, inflammatory joint changes, and damaged cartilage.

9. Arthrocentesis is the procedure used to obtain fluid from a joint.
10. Normal phosphorus levels are 1.7–2.6 mEq/L or 2.5–4.5 mg/dL. Phosphorus has an inverse relationship with calcium. When calcium levels are up, phosphorus will be down, and vice versa.

## Apply What You Learned

1. The nurse assesses and documents muscle strength, grading muscle strength from 0 to 5, with 0 being no muscle contraction or paralysis and 5 being full range of motion against resistance. Evaluating specific muscle groups can be done, for example, by asking the patient to close her eyes tightly to check eye and lid strength; blow out her cheeks and stick out her tongue to check facial muscles; hold her arms up to check deltoids; and bend and straighten her arms to check biceps and triceps.

2. The nurse assesses range of motion when he inspects and palpates bones and joints. It is important to assess and compare corresponding joints on both sides of the body. Joints such as the shoulders and knees are palpated for crepitus. Evaluating specific joints for ROM can be done, for example, by asking the patient to put his chin to his chest to check for cervical spine flexion; look at the ceiling to check for cervical spine extension; touch his toes with his fingers to check for lumbar spine flexion; slowly bend backward to check for lumbar spine expansion; and raise his arms straight out to the side to check for shoulder abduction.

## Multiple Choice

| | | | |
|---|---|---|---|
| 1. | D | 9. | B |
| 2. | B | 10. | A |
| 3. | A | 11. | B |
| 4. | B | 12. | A |
| 5. | C | 13. | B |
| 6. | D | 14. | C |
| 7. | B | 15. | A |
| 8. | C | | |

## Chapter 42   Caring for Patients with Musculoskeletal Trauma

## Matching

| | | | |
|---|---|---|---|
| 1. | J | 6. | H |
| 2. | C | 7. | F |
| 3. | G | 8. | B |
| 4. | I | 9. | E |
| 5. | A | 10. | D |

## Learning Outcomes

1. Characteristics of a sprain include ligament injury, joint instability, pain, swelling, discoloration, and increased pain with joint use.

2. With a closed (simple) fracture, the skin over the fracture remains intact. With an open (compound) fracture, broken bone protrudes through the skin. With a comminuted fracture, bone fragments into many pieces. With a compression fracture, bone is crushed. With an impacted fracture, broken ends of bone are forced together. With a depressed fracture, broken bone is pressed inward. With a spiral fracture, a jagged break occurs due to twisting force. With a greenstick fracture, an incomplete break occurs along the length of the bone.

3. Compartment syndrome occurs when excess pressure restricts blood vessels and nerves within a compartment. It may be caused by bleeding or edema within the compartment or by external compression of the limb by a too-tight cast.

4. Carpal tunnel syndrome is one of the most common work-related injuries. The carpal tunnel is a can through which tendons and the median nerve pass from the wrist to the hand. The syndrome develops when the tunnel narrows, compressing and irritating the median nerve. This usually results from inflammation and swelling of structures in the wrist joint.

5. Phantom pain is felt along nerves of the body part that has been amputated. The exact cause is unknown, but it may be caused by trauma to the nerves serving the amputated part. The missing extremity feels numb, crushed, trapped, twisted, or burning. Management is challenging and often requires referral to a pain clinic.

6. To decrease fractures in older adults, monitor responses to medications, introduce assistive devices in stages as reflexes slow and gait alterations appear, address safety issues such as risks for falling, assess the need for in-home assistance, and make appropriate referrals to visiting nurses and home health aides.

7. Manual traction is applied by physically pulling the extremity. It is often used to reduce a fracture or dislocation. Skin traction applies the pulling force through the patient's skin. Balanced suspension traction uses more than one force of pull to raise and support the injured extremity off the bed and maintain its alignment. In skeletal traction, the pulling force is applied directly through pins inserted into the bone.

8. Manifestations of compartment syndrome include pain, pallor, paresthesias, paresis, and pulselessness.

9. Fat emboli occur when fat globules lodge in a pulmonary vessel or the peripheral circulation. In the bloodstream, fat globules combine with platelets and travel to the brain, lungs, kidneys, and other organs, blocking small vessels and causing tissue ischemia.

10. RICE is an acronym used to remember initial measures to treat soft tissue trauma. The goal is to decrease swelling, alleviate pain, and encourage rest and healing. RICE stands for Rest, Ice, Compression, and Elevation.

## Apply What You Learned

1. Encourage verbalization and validation of feelings. Contact the physician for a referral to a psychologist or social worker. Teach the importance of moving and ROM exercises to prevent contractures. Also encourage turning and lying in the prone position.

2. The nurse can contact social services to assist the patient with home health nurses and financial resources. The nurse should also contact the dietician to ensure the patient is getting what he needs to promote wound healing.

## Multiple Choice

1. C
2. D
3. B
4. C
5. A
6. B
7. B
8. A
9. C
10. C
11. C
12. A
13. A
14. B
15. C

## Matching

1. E
2. F
3. G
4. H
5. D

6. B
7. C
8. I
9. A
10. J

## Learning Outcomes

1. Complications of osteoporosis include loss of height, progressive curvature of the spine, low back pain, and fractures.

2. In osteomyelitis, pathogens usually enter the bone through an open wound, such as an open fracture or a gunshot or puncture wound. Bacteria may also spread to the bone from a local tissue infection. After entry, bacteria lodge and multiply in the bone, causing an inflammatory and immune system response. Phagocytes attempt to contain the infection. In the process, they release enzymes that destroy bone tissue. Pus forms, followed by edema and vascular congestion. Canals in the marrow cavity of the bone allow the infection to spread to other parts of the bone. If the infection reaches the outer margin of the bone, it raises the periosteum of the bone and spreads along the surface. Pus and edema disrupt the blood supply to the bone, leading to ischemia and, eventually, necrosis of the bone.

3. Osteoarthritis is a degenerative joint disease characterized by progressive loss of joint cartilage in synovial joints. It is the most common type of arthritis and is a leading cause of disability in older adults.

4. Rheumatoid arthritis is a chronic, systemic inflammatory disorder that primarily affects the joints. It is a connective tissue disorder that affects more women than men and usually develops between the ages of 30 and 50.

5. Lupus erythematosus is a chronic inflammatory connective tissue disease. It affects multiple body systems and can range in severity from mild and episodic to a rapidly fatal disease. A cardinal sign of lupus is the butterfly rash on the face.

6. Fibromyalgia is a common rheumatic syndrome of musculoskeletal pain, stiffness, and tenderness.

7. Although patients of all backgrounds are at risk for developing osteoporosis, ethnicity affects risk. Among women age 50 and older, non-Hispanic White and Asian women have the highest risk. One in 10 Hispanic women is affected by osteoporosis, and nearly half have low bone mass. Black women have a lower incidence, with 1 in 20 affected by osteoporosis and just over one-third with low bone mass.

8. Multisystem effects of lupus include butterfly rash on face, alopecia, depression, renal failure, photophobia, anemia, arthralgias, anorexia, pleurisy, dementia, and vasculitis.

9. Manifestations of rheumatoid arthritis include swelling, warmth, tenderness, and pain in the joints; limited range of motion and morning stiffness that lasts more than one hour; joint destruction; and deformity including nodules over the elbows, joints, and toes.

10. Arthralgia is localized joint pain and is the most common symptom of OA.

## Apply What You Learned

1. Discharge teaching for this patient would include providing him with a list, including pictures, of the exercises and ROM he is permitted to do. Referrals to home health and physical therapy along with a follow-up appointment with the surgeon should be scheduled in a timely manner to decrease complications. The patient should be taught about pain control and when to call the physician.

2. Ask the patient and his wife to recall the information that was reviewed with them. Ask them to demonstrate the exercises as well as what information they need when they call the physician.

## Multiple Choice

1. A
2. D
3. C
4. A
5. C
6. C
7. D
8. D
9. B
10. D
11. A
12. C
13. C
14. B
15. D

## Chapter 44   The Integumentary System and Assessment

## Matching

1. G
2. D
3. J
4. I
5. B
6. E
7. H
8. C
9. F
10. A

## Learning Outcomes

1. The epidermis protects tissues from physical, chemical, and biologic damage; prevents water loss and serves as a water-repellent layer; stores melanin; converts cholesterol molecules to vitamin D when exposed to sunlight; and contains phagocytes, which prevent bacteria from penetrating the skin.

2. The dermis regulates body temperature by dilating and constricting capillaries and transmits messag via nerve endings to the CNS.

3. Three types of glands in the skin are sebaceous (oil), eccrine sweat glands, and apocrine sweat glands.

4. A vesicle is an elevated, fluid-filled, round- or oval-shaped, palpable mass with thin, translucent walls and circumscribed borders. Vesicles are smaller than 0.5 cm.

5. A keloid occurs from a scar related to surgery or ear piercing. It is an elevated, irregular, darkened area of excess scar tissue caused by excessive collagen formation during healing. There is a higher incidence of keloids in people of African descent.

6. Clubbing is an angle of the nail base that is greater than 180 degrees.

7. A biopsy is done when a sample of a nodule or skin is needed to rule out malignancy. It can be done with a syringe to pull out fluid or with a special biopsy instrument.

8. A culture and sensitivity (C&S) is done when fluid obtained from bullae, pustules, or abscesses is thought to have a bacterial or viral infection.

9. Suspected allergens are applied to normal skin under patches. Reactions range from weak with redness or itching, to strong with pain and blisters.

10. The color of the skin is the result of varying levels of pigmentation. Melanin is darker and is produced in greater amounts in persons with dark skin color than in those with light skin. Exposure to the sun causes a buildup of melanin and a darkening of the skin in people with light skin. Carotene is more abundant in the skins of persons of Asian ancestry, and together with melanin accounts for their golden skin tone. The epidermis in Caucasian skin has very little melanin and is almost transparent. The color of their red blood cells shows through, lending Caucasians a pinkish skin tone. Skin color is influenced by emotions and illnesses; for example, erythema, cyanosis, pallor, or jaundice may be the result of various emotions or illnesses.

## Apply What You Learned

1. The nurse should discuss that a variety of normal skin changes are seen in the older adult. Loss of subcutaneous tissue, dermal thinning, and decreased elasticity may cause wrinkles and sagging of the skin. The skin is thinner, and turgor is decreased. Older adults are unable to respond to heat or cold quickly, increasing their risk for heat stroke and hypothermia. In addition, the older adult may experience dry, itchy skin as a result of the reduced number of sweat and oil glands; decreased overall production of melanocytes and abnormal localized proliferations of melanocytes in specific areas; skin tags; decreased hair and nail growth; gray hair; and thickened, yellowed, and peeling nails.

2. Primary and secondary skin lesions to be aware of are macules and patches, nodules and tumors, papules and plaques, vesicles and bullae, wheals, scales, pustules, crusts, cysts, ulcers, atrophy, fissures, erosion, scars, lichenification, and keloids.

## Multiple Choice

1. C
2. D
3. A
4. C
5. B
6. D
7. A
8. D
9. D
10. B
11. A
12. A
13. C
14. B
15. C

## Chapter 45    Caring for Patients with Skin Disorders

## Matching

1. F
2. J
3. D
4. G
5. E
6. H
7. B
8. A
9. I
10. C

## Learning Outcomes

1. Psoriasis is a chronic, noninfectious skin disorder. It is characterized by raised, reddened, round circumscribed plaques of varied size, covered by silvery-white scales.

2. Contact dermatitis is caused by a hypersensitivity response or a chemical irritation. Major sources include perfumes, dyes, plants, metals, and chemicals.

3. Cellulitis is a localized infection of the dermis and subcutaneous tissue. It can occur following a wound or skin ulcer.

4. Folliculitis begins at the skin surface and extends down into the hair follicle. It is most often caused by *Staphylococcus aureus*. The bacteria release enzymes and chemical agents that cause an inflammation.

5. Basal cell carcinoma is a slow-growing cancer that usually appears on sun-exposed areas of the body, such as the head and neck. These carcinomas can recur in the same location after treatment. They have a shiny, pearly white, or pink appearance in nodular carcinoma. The superficial carcinomas are a flat papule that is often red.

6. Steps to prevent skin cancer include the following: minimize exposure to the sun between the hours of 10 a.m. and 4 p.m. when the ultraviolet rays are the strongest; wear a wide-brimmed hat, sunglasses, and a long woven shirt when you are in the sun; use sunscreen and remember to reapply; and avoid tanning booths.

7. Pressure ulcers are ischemic lesions of the skin and underlying tissue caused by external pressure that impairs the flow of blood and lymph. The ischemia causes tissue necrosis and eventual ulceration.

8. Pressure ulcer stages are as follows: Stage I is nonblanchable erythema of a localized area intact skin. Stage II is partial-thickness loss of dermis. Stage III is full-thickness tissue loss; subcutaneous fat may be visible, but bone, tendon, or muscle are not exposed, and undermining and tunneling may be present. Stage IV is full-thickness tissue loss with exposed bone, tendon, or muscle; often includes undermining and tunneling.

9. Melanoma is a skin cancer that causes 4% of all skin cancer cases. The incidence is highest in Caucasians; people who had severe, blistering sunburns during childhood; and in people who live in sunny climates, burn easily, and visit tanning booths. They also may arise from lesions that are already present or from skin that is normally covered with clothing. Melanomas start off flat, but with progression into the lymph, they become raised.

10. Nevi are moles and the precursor for the development of melanoma.

## Apply What You Learned

1. To self-screen for skin cancer, the patient follows the ABCDE rule: A is for asymmetry of the mole; B is for border irregularity; C is for color variation; D is for diameter greater than 5 mm; and E is for evolution (history of skin lesion changing).

2. This patient presented with basal cell carcinoma.

3. The patient should wear sunscreen even in the tanning booth. She should try to avoid the sun between 10 a.m. and 4 p.m. as well as avoid the tanning beds. The patient should wear wide-brimmed hats and sunglasses when in the sun. She should also protect exposed arms and legs with woven clothing.

## Multiple Choice

| | | | |
|---|---|---|---|
| 1. | A | 9. | B |
| 2. | B | 10. | C |
| 3. | C | 11. | B |
| 4. | C | 12. | A |
| 5. | C | 13. | C |
| 6. | D | 14. | A |
| 7. | D | 15. | C |
| 8. | C | | |

## Chapter 46  Caring for Patients with Burns

## Matching

| | | | |
|---|---|---|---|
| 1. | F | 6. | J |
| 2. | D | 7. | B |
| 3. | A | 8. | E |
| 4. | I | 9. | C |
| 5. | G | 10. | H |

## Learning Outcomes

1. Thermal burns result from exposure to dry heat or moist heat. They are the most common burns and occur mostly in children and older adults. Chemical burns are caused by direct skin contact with either acid or alkaline agents. The severity of electrical burns depends on the type and duration of current and amount of voltage. Electricity follows the path of lease resistance, which in the human body tends to lie along muscles, blood vessels, nerves, and bone.

2. The "rule of nines" is a rapid method of estimating the extent of burns. It is used during prehospital and emergency care phases.
3. Curling ulcer is an acute ulceration of the stomach or duodenum that may form following a burn injury.
4. Debridement is the process of removing dead tissue from the wound.
5. Initial assessments regarding burns include time of injury, cause, first-aid treatment, past medical history, age, medications, and body weight.
6. Nursing diagnoses related to the burn patient include Deficient Fluid Volume, Risk for Infection, Impaired Physical Mobility, Acute Pain, and Powerlessness.
7. Both types of dressing are applied after the wound has been cleaned and debrided. In the open method of wound dressing, the burn remains open to air, covered only by a topical antimicrobial agent. Strict isolation precautions must be followed, and topical agents are reapplied frequently because they tend to rub off onto the bedding. In the closed method, a topical antimicrobial agent is applied to the wound site, which is covered with gauze or a nonadherent dressing and then gently wrapped with a gauze roll bandage. Wounds with closed dressings are usually dressed twice daily and as needed.
8. The silver nitrate solution is applied to gauze dressings every 2 hours, and dressings are changed completely twice a day. The patient must be monitored for decreased serum sodium and chloride levels because large amounts of water are absorbed from the dressing site. The patient should be taught that silver nitrate causes the skin and dressings to turn black. The patient should report symptoms of infection, swelling, weight gain, or breathing difficulty.
9. Urinalysis, CBC, serum electrolytes, total protein and albumin, ABGs, pulse oximetry, CXR, and ECGs are tests done to monitor and assess burns.
10. Patient and family teaching are an important component of all phases of burn care. As treatment progresses, the nurse should encourage family members to assume more responsibility in providing care. From admission to discharge, the nurse should teach the patient and family to assess all findings, implement therapies, and evaluate progress. It should be emphasized that the goal of all care is to prevent soft tissue deformity, protect skin grafts, maintain physiologic function, manage scars, and return the patient to his or her optimal level of independence. The teaching plan focuses on helping the patient and family prevent dehydration, infection, and pain; maintain adequate nutrition and skin integrity; and restore mobility and psychosocial well-being.

## Apply What You Learned

1. 4 ½% of his body is burned. Remember that the rule of nines is just an estimate.
2. Silvadene would be used on this patient to prevent burn wound infections. This patient may also see a plastic surgeon throughout the healing process to identify if corrective surgery is needed.

## Multiple Choice

| | |
|---|---|
| 1. B | 9. C |
| 2. D | 10. A |
| 3. C | 11. D |
| 4. C | 12. A |
| 5. A | 13. C |
| 6. B | 14. B |
| 7. A | 15. C |
| 8. A | |

## Matching

| | | | |
|---|---|---|---|
| 1. | D | 6. | G |
| 2. | F | 7. | I |
| 3. | A | 8. | B |
| 4. | C | 9. | J |
| 5. | H | 10. | E |

## Learning Outcomes

1. Aspects of a mentally healthy person are an accurate assessment of reality, healthy self-concept, ability to relate to others, sense of meaning in life, creativity/abstract thinking, productivity or contribution to the benefit of others, control over one's behavior, and an adaptability to change and conflict.

2. Insight is important because it allows people to see their own motivations or reasons behind their feelings and behavior. Insight is critical for problem solving; without it, people often do not realize that they have a mental illness.

3. Neurotransmitters include acetylcholine, dopamine, norepinephrine, serotonin, and GABA.

4. A synapse is the space between the axon and its target cell's dendrite.

5. Mental illness has a stigma in our culture, which can deter affected people from seeking the treatment they need, even when that treatment can save lives. Even physicians sometimes hesitate to give their patients the diagnosis of a mental disorder for fear that the patients will be "labeled" and treated badly as a result. Negative labels for people with mental illness are inaccurate, inappropriate, and ignorant. As patient advocates, nurses should stop using these negative labels and educate the public that mental illnesses should be treated in the same way as physical illnesses.

6. Psychologic functions include thinking, feeling, behavior, responses to situations, relationships, and community support.

7. Four aspects of self-concept are body image, role performance, identity, and self-esteem.

8. The five most common mental illnesses are major depressive disorder, alcohol abuse, schizophrenia, self-inflicted injuries, and bipolar disorder.

9. Mental illnesses are diagnosed according to the diagnostic criteria published in the *Diagnostic and Statistical Manual of Mental Disorders*.

10. Risk factors related to mental illness include inability to reach developmental tasks, hopelessness, imbalance of brain neurotransmitters, lack of information about treatment options, inadequate role models for values and behaviour, inadequate coping skills, inadequate resources, substance dependency, exhaustion, extreme stress, and a genetic predisposition to mental illness.

## Apply What You Learned

1. Elements of a complete mental status assessment are appearance, orientation to surroundings, mood and affect, speech, thoughts, hallucinations, behavior, memory, and judgment.

2. "What happened that caused you to come to the hospital?" It is straightforward and nonjudgmental.

## Multiple Choice

| | | | |
|---|---|---|---|
| 1. | B | 9. | A |
| 2. | B | 10. | C |
| 3. | B | 11. | A |
| 4. | A | 12. | C |
| 5. | C | 13. | B |
| 6. | D | 14. | A |
| 7. | C | 15. | C |
| 8. | A | | |

# Chapter 48   Caring for Patients with Neurocognitive Disorders

## Matching

1. J
2. B
3. F
4. A
5. C

6. H
7. D
8. G
9. E
10. I

## Learning Outcomes

1. Normal memory lapses may include forgetting where you left your keys or wallet, searching to find a word that is on the tip of your tongue, and losing track of what you planned to say.
2. Delirium may manifest either with motor agitation or motor retardation, sudden onset of severe agitation and hallucinations, or declining level of consciousness progressing to coma.
3. The MMSE consists of questions related to orientation, registration, attention and calculation, recall, and language, for a total score of 30 points.
4. Agnosia is the loss of comprehension of visual, auditory, or other sensations, although the sensory structures are intact.
5. Common causes of dementia include neurodegenerative disorders, vascular-based disorders, metabolic diseases, immunologic diseases, infections, tumors, and seizures.
6. Alzheimer disease is a neurologic disorder in which neurofibrillary tangles and beta-amyloid plaques cause deterioration of brain function, characterized by a progressive loss of memory.
7. Risk factors for vascular dementia include advanced age, hypertension, hyperlipidemia, atrial fibrillation, coronary artery disease, and diabetes.
8. Delirium has a quick onset, is worse at night, includes sleep disturbances, and is temporary. Dementia has a gradual onset and symptoms progress slowly. The patient frequently awakens in the night. It is chronic with a life expectancy after diagnosis of 8 years.
9. Delirium is associated with a variety of general medical conditions, surgery, polypharmacy, infections, drugs, alcohol, and severe psychosocial stressors. Dementia is related to neurodegenerative disorders, vascular abnormalities, toxic or metabolic disorders, immune abnormalities, infections, systemic diseases, seizure disorders, low pressure hydrocephalus, and drugs. Depression is a brain neurotransmitter deficit.
10. Medications used to treat dementia are Aricept, Exelon, Razadyne, Namenda, and Cognex.

## Apply What You Learned

1. The above characteristics indicate onset of Alzheimer disease.
2. Following the physician's diagnosis, the patient should be started on medication to slow the progression of dementia. Senior centers, home nurses, and perhaps a Meals on Wheels program would be beneficial for this patient. A senior center might ensure the patient is socially active and not becoming withdrawn. Home care nurses can make certain the patient is taking medication and is safe at home, and Meals on Wheels can ensure the patient has an appropriate diet.
3. Nursing diagnoses for this patient would include Risk for Injury related to impaired judgment and disorientation, Disturbed Thought Processes, Language Deficit, and Deficient Knowledge.

## Multiple Choice

| | | | |
|---|---|---|---|
| 1. | B | 9. | D |
| 2. | D | 10. | D |
| 3. | A | 11. | C |
| 4. | C | 12. | B |
| 5. | A | 13. | B |
| 6. | D | 14. | A |
| 7. | A | 15. | D |
| 8. | B | | |

## Chapter 49　Caring for Patients with Psychotic Disorders

### Matching

| | | | |
|---|---|---|---|
| 1. | G | 6. | J |
| 2. | B | 7. | I |
| 3. | F | 8. | D |
| 4. | A | 9. | H |
| 5. | E | 10. | C |

### Learning Outcomes

1. Psychosis refers to a thought disorder that causes the following symptoms: delusions, hallucinations, disorganized speech, and disorganized behavior.
2. A hallucination is a sensory experience that seems real to the patient but is not related to external stimuli. The most common hallucinations are auditory; the second most common are visual. Hallucinations can involve any of the senses.
3. Schizophrenia is the most common thought disorder.
4. Manifestations of schizophrenia may include delusions, hallucinations, disorganized speech, grossly disorganized or catatonic behaviour, and/or negative symptoms, as well as seriously impaired self-care, social, or occupational function. The duration of symptoms must be at least 6 months, and the symptoms must not be caused by another disorder or drugs.
5. For psychiatric inpatients, the environment, or milieu, can be used as part of therapy. It should be pleasant, simple, and safe. There should be minimal stimulation and consistent nursing staff. Reminders are given about self-care, and group activities are planned to promote health. This type of therapy provides structure for patients' daily living.
6. Nursing diagnoses for patients with psychotic disorders include Risk for Violence, Disturbed Thought Processes, Ineffective Coping, and Impaired Social Interaction.
7. Outcomes for a patient with schizophrenia include cause no harm to self or others, have reality-based thinking, use healthy coping skills, take medications regularly, and keep in touch with family and friends.
8. Neuroleptic malignant syndrome is a potentially fatal side effect of antipsychotic drugs. The major symptoms are high fever, muscle rigidity, autonomic instability, delirium, inability to speak, tremors, and elevated levels of enzymes that indicate muscle damage.
9. During the prodromal phase, the patient has early symptoms before a full psychotic episode.
10. A patient with bizarre delusions believes clearly improbable ideas that are not derived from real-life experiences.

## Apply What You Learned

1. This patient might receive a diagnosis of schizophrenia.
2. Only one person should interact with the patient at a time to prevent overstimulation. Keep environmental noise to a minimum and do not speak loudly. This will enable the patient to concentrate on your voice and differentiate real stimuli from the nonreal stimuli. Initially ask about the hallucination so that a determination can be made if there is an intent to commit harm. Focus on reality. Do not ask the patient to continually describe the hallucination. Bring the patient back to reality as often as necessary without getting the patient agitated. Do not argue with the patient's experience. Reassure the patient that he or she is safe. Share your own perceptions by letting the patient know that you do not hear any voices. Avoid touching the patient if the patient is actively hallucinating. The patient may see this as a threat, and the goal is safety for the patient and staff.

## Multiple Choice

| | | | |
|---|---|---|---|
| 1. | C | 9. | A |
| 2. | A | 10. | A |
| 3. | B | 11. | A |
| 4. | B | 12. | B |
| 5. | D | 13. | D |
| 6. | D | 14. | A |
| 7. | C | 15. | A |
| 8. | B | | |

## Chapter 50   Caring for Patients with Mood Disorders

## Matching

| | | | |
|---|---|---|---|
| 1. | D | 6. | B |
| 2. | C | 7. | J |
| 3. | A | 8. | E |
| 4. | G | 9. | F |
| 5. | I | 10. | H |

## Learning Outcomes

1. Mood can be elevated, with an exaggerated sense of energy or well-being; euthymic, which is in the normal range; dysphoric, which is sad or unpleasant; or irritable, a mood in which one is easily annoyed, upset, or provoked to anger.
2. Risk factors for depression include family history, female gender, stressful life events, substance abuse, postpartum period, chronic medical condition, and history of a suicide attempt.
3. Psychomotor agitation is an increase in activity.
4. Protective factors for suicide are effective and appropriate clinical care, easy access to support, family support, and learned skills in problem solving and conflict resolution.
5. Suicide is the taking of one's own life.
6. Anticholinergic side effects include dry mouth, increased heart rate, constipation, pupil dilation, blurred near vision, dry eyes, and photophobia.
7. Foods to avoid when taking MAOIs are those that are high in tyramine, including aged cheese, preserved meats, liver, draft beer, soy sauce, yeast, and caffeine.

8. ECT is the application of electrical current to the brain, which induces a generalized seizure. The exact mechanism of action is not known, but ECT does increase circulating levels of brain neurotransmitters, which may be the way it relieves depression. ECT is used for patients who have intense, prolonged symptoms with marked disability, especially if the patient has not responded to adequate trial with medications or if psychotic features are present.

9. While manic, the patient feels elated, euphoric, high, or unusually good. People in a manic episode frequently lack insight about their illness and its effects on themselves and others. They often resist treatment and sometimes require involuntary hospitalization. Periods of mania alternate with periods of depression.

10. The nurse should teach the patient taking lithium that dehydration and NSAIDs increase the risk of toxicity due to increased Li levels; that high Na intake increases Li excretion, so the patient should maintain stable (or reduce) Na intake and replace losses due to sweating; that blood tests for Li levels are necessary throughout treatment; symptoms of toxicity; and the importance of properly using contraceptives.

## Apply What You Learned

1. Use open-ended questions when asking the patient to express feelings. Clarify the patient's statements. Gather data for assessment and validate the patient's feelings. Obtain a "no self-harm" contract and assess the patient's current safety.

2. "Are you thinking about hurting yourself?"

## Multiple Choice

| | | | |
|---|---|---|---|
| 1. | D | 9. | D |
| 2. | A | 10. | C |
| 3. | C | 11. | A |
| 4. | B | 12. | B |
| 5. | D | 13. | C |
| 6. | A | 14. | A |
| 7. | C | 15. | D |
| 8. | B | | |

## Chapter 51    Caring for Patients with Anxiety Disorders

## Matching

| | | | |
|---|---|---|---|
| 1. | C | 6. | A |
| 2. | I | 7. | H |
| 3. | B | 8. | F |
| 4. | E | 9. | G |
| 5. | J | 10. | D |

## Learning Outcomes

1. Feelings, physiologic responses, and thoughts are all part of the anxiety experience. During anxiety, there is an increase in blood flow to the limbic system and the cerebral cortex. The limbic system conducts stimuli to the sympathetic part of the ANS. Sympathetic stimulation causes the symptoms we recognize as anxiety. From the limbic system, neural messages are also conducted to the cerebral cortex. In the association areas of the cerebral cortex, the individual experiences thoughts about anxiety.

2. Manifestations of panic attacks include palpitations, sweating, trembling, feeling of choking, chest pain, nausea, feeling dizzy, and fear of losing control.

3. PTSD is a debilitating condition that follows an extreme traumatic stressor such as a violent personal attack or war.

4. Medical conditions associated with anxiety are hypoglycemia, asthma, COPD, B12 deficiency, hyperthyroidism, and neoplasms.

5. Defense mechanisms include acting out, altruism, anticipation, compensation, denial, displacement, dissociation, humor, intellectualization, projection, rationalization, reaction formation, regression, repression, sublimation, and suppression.

6. Resilience is the quality of being hardy, and several resilience factors are self-efficacy, regular exercise, high functional ability, independence with ADLs, good self-rated health, and positive outlook on life.

7. Antianxiety agents include Xanax, Librium, Klonopin, Valium, Ativan, Serax, and Tranxene.

8. Expected outcomes related to a patient with anxiety include that he or she will discuss feelings of anxiety and potential desire to harm self; will verbalize strategies to interrupt anxiety; and will discuss feelings and verbalize situations that increase the sense of threat, fear, or anxiety.

9. OCD is characterized by compulsions or obsessions, which the affected person recognizes are excessive or unreasonable. The obsessions or compulsions cause marked distress and take more than 1 hour each day, or significantly interfere with the person's life.

10. Social anxiety disorder is characterized by a marked and persistent fear of social or performance situations in which embarrassment may occur.

## Apply What You Learned

1. The nurse would expect a diagnosis of posttraumatic stress disorder.

2. This patient would benefit from learning coping techniques, cognitive-behavior therapy, promoting resilience, and the use of medication and regular therapy sessions with a licensed professional.

## Multiple Choice

1. A
2. C
3. C
4. D
5. C
6. B
7. C
8. C
9. D
10. D
11. A
12. D
13. A
14. C
15. A

## Chapter 52   Caring for Patients with Personality Disorders

## Matching

1. C
2. D
3. G
4. H
5. F
6. E
7. I
8. J
9. B
10. A

## Learning Outcomes

1. The five basic personality traits are extroversion, agreeableness, conscientiousness, emotional stability, and openness.

2. Cluster A is odd and eccentric, Cluster B is dramatic and emotional, and Cluster C is anxiety- and fear-based.

3. A patient with inappropriate affect has emotional responses that are not culturally appropriate for particular situations, such as laughing when someone's pet dies. The thinking, behavior, speech, and appearance of affected people are also likely to be eccentric or peculiar. These patients will probably not have friends, and they have excessive social anxiety that does not resolve as people become more familiar.

4. APD is a pervasive pattern of disregarding and violating the rights of others.
5. A narcissistic person has a need for admiration, patterns of grandiosity, and lack of empathy for others. They have an inflated sense of self and feel entitled.
6. Patients with dependent personality disorder have a need to be taken care of. They have submissive and clinging behavior. They have difficulty making everyday decisions without help and advice from others.
7. Coping mechanisms for a patient who suffers from self-harm are talking to someone, delaying your decision for 5 minutes, calling a crisis line, yelling, screaming, crying, singing loudly, or pounding on your bed until you are exhausted.
8. Borderline personality disorder describes patients who are on the border between anxiety and psychosis.
9. The priority short-term goal for patients with antisocial personality is to prevent harm to self or others. This patient may be manipulative and physically violent, so these issues should be managed first. Other goals include anger management, coping skills, increasing self-awareness, and learning to see an event from another person's point of view. Group therapy may help. The staff must cooperate to consistently apply the treatment plan and facility policies.
10. For a patient with disturbed thought processes, interventions include not ignoring the patient's suspicions but at the same time not overemphasizing his or her fears; approaching the patient with a matter-of-fact, professional attitude; reassuring the patient that he or she is safe and that the staff is making every effort to provide accurate, quality care; adhering strictly to the rules of the organization; and trying some corrective statements.

## *Apply What You Learned*

1. Make the unit rules clear. Policies must be maintained. Stick to the rules consistently. Include the patient in problem solving and have a conference with him or her. Remember who is the patient and who is the professional.
2. The nurse should make brief and nonthreatening interpersonal interactions with the patient, provide low-stress opportunity for the patient to be with other people, and provide some social skills training.

## *Multiple Choice*

| | | | |
|---|---|---|---|
| 1. C | | 9. C | |
| 2. B | | 10. C | |
| 3. A | | 11. A | |
| 4. A | | 12. B | |
| 5. A | | 13. A | |
| 6. D | | 14. A | |
| 7. C | | 15. C | |
| 8. B | | | |

## Chapter 53    Caring for Patients with Substance Use Disorders

## *Matching*

| | | | |
|---|---|---|---|
| 1. G | | 6. A | |
| 2. H | | 7. C | |
| 3. F | | 8. E | |
| 4. I | | 9. D | |
| 5. J | | 10. B | |

## Learning Outcomes

1. Denial is the refusal to acknowledge the existence of a real situation or feelings. It is a common coping mechanism for people with substance use disorders and for the health professionals who work with them.
2. Commonly abused substances include alcohol, opioids, sedatives, cocaine, hallucinogens, inhalants, caffeine, and nicotine.
3. Someone withdrawing from alcohol may have elevated vital signs, anxiety, tremors, diaphoresis, slurred speech, GI disturbances, and disorientation.
4. Korsakoff syndrome is a group of symptoms caused by a deficiency in the B vitamins, including thiamine, riboflavin, and folic acid.
5. Wernicke syndrome is characterized by ataxia, paralysis of the eye muscles, and mental confusion. It is the result of severe vitamin B1 deficiency from lack of adequate nutritional intake.
6. Fetal alcohol syndrome presents with low birth weight, small head circumference, facial anomalies, and neurodevelopmental disorders.
7. Detoxification is the removal of a substance from the body.
8. Rehabilitation is a continuous phase related to substance abuse. Medications and therapies, as well as support groups, are utilized to prevent relapses for the rest of the patient's life. The goals of rehab are to maintain sobriety, develop new coping skills, make a plan for relapse prevention and living life with all responsibilities, and be able to cope effectively.
9. Dual diagnosis refers to someone who is diagnosed with a substance use disorder and a serious mental illness.
10. An impaired nurse is someone who is working under the influence of substances. He or she may exhibit mood changes, irritability, forgetfulness, and isolation from coworkers. In addition, work performance may suffer.

## Apply What You Learned

1. Stereotypes related to alcoholics include lack of education, low socioeconomic background, non-Caucasian ethnicity, and unemployment. Everyone, regardless of status and position in life, is susceptible to alcoholism.
2. The student nurse would begin by asking the patient how much and how often he or she drinks. The nurse will also ask the patient about the use of any nonprescribed drugs and for what purpose. The student nurse also needs to ask what these substances do for the patient, that is, what benefit they provide. Also, the nurse needs to try to identify any problems the patient has been having since using any substance. The patient should also be questioned about the last time they used a substance and what it was.

## Multiple Choice

| | | | |
|---|---|---|---|
| 1. | C | 9. | C |
| 2. | B | 10. | D |
| 3. | D | 11. | D |
| 4. | A | 12. | A |
| 5. | A | 13. | C |
| 6. | C | 14. | C |
| 7. | C | 15. | D |
| 8. | B | | |